An honest and unabashed look at how Paula faced one of life's most fearful battles with an inner strength, self-determination and boundless faith, bolstered by her husband Jack's unwavering love and support, to conquer convention and an oft-times unconquerable foe. An important read for anyone. Dennis C. Duffy, Fellow Writer

This book is a must read for anyone fighting cancer since it's an invaluable resource filled with a wealth of information and experience. Although Paula's healing journey began conventionally, she courageously pursued unconventional and alternative methods. While this is a compelling story of healing, it's also the epitome of the 1 Corinthians 13:13 verse about faith, hope and love; because the heart of this book is a true love story. Denita Stevens, Writer and Poet

Whether you or a loved one is battling cancer, or even a skeptic to alternative treatments, Guided Cure is a compelling journey of overcoming cancer through holistic healing. Paula's story combines physical healing with spiritual, emotional and psychological healing—teaching us to question every treatment and leave no stone unturned. A provocative approach told with humor, faith, love and a tenacity for the right answers. Donna Powell, Skeptic turned believer.

Paula Beiger's "Guided Cure" is a journey through the physical, metaphysical, dreadful, and hysterical story of her own personal bout with cancer. You will laugh. You will cry. You will be introduced to a myriad of alternative therapies and treatments that you'll have no choice but to open your mind to. It is a story of hope, recovery, and family – a quick read and a blessing for anyone considering alternative care! Dr. Eric Jaszewski, DC

D0200314

Guided
Cure

A Healing Memoir

By Paula Beiger

Foreword by Mark James Bartiss, MD

DISCLAIMER: The techniques and suggestions expressed here are intended to be used for educational purposes only. We are not rendering medical advice, nor to diagnose, prescribe or treat any disease, condition or illness. It is recommended that before beginning any nutrition or exercise program you received clearance from your physician. I have tried to recreate events and conversations from my memories of them. In some instances, the names of individuals and places have been changed to protect the privacy of the individuals.

First edition printed December 2016

ISBN 13: 978 1540851758
ISBN 10: 1540851753

Cover Design by
Paula & Jack Beiger

Edited by
Paula Plantier
EditAmerica

Table of Contents

Ecclesiastes
3: 1-13

1 To every thing there is a season, and a time to every purpose under the heaven:

2 A time to be born, and a time to die; a time to plant, and a time to pluck up that which is planted;

3 A time to kill, and a time to heal; a time to break down, and a time to build up;

4 A time to weep, and a time to laugh; a time to mourn, and a time to dance;

5 A time to cast away stones, and a time to gather stones together; a time to embrace, and a time to refrain from embracing;

6 A time to get, and a time to lose; a time to keep, and a time to cast away;

7 A time to rend, and a time to sew; a time to keep silence, and a time to speak;

8 A time to love, and a time to hate; a time of war, and a time of peace.

9 What profit hath he that worketh in that wherein he laboureth?

10 I have seen the travail, which God hath given to the sons of men to be exercised in it.

11 He hath made every thing beautiful in his time: also he hath set the world in their heart, so that no man can find out the work that God maketh from the beginning to the end.

12 I know that there is no good in them, but for a man to rejoice, and to do good in his life.

13 And also that every man should eat and drink, and enjoy the good of all his labour, it is the gift of God.

DEDICATION

This book is dedicated to the two Rhodas in my life. The first is my mother, Eileen Rhoda Kennedy Quackenboss. The second is my mom's namesake great granddaughter, Rhoda-Jane Louise Taylor.

My mom passed away from lung cancer at the age of 74. There was an inoperable tumor on her lung.

My mom was always a character.

When the doctors told her they could prolong her life a few months if she agreed to chemotherapy and radiation, she said, "I don't want to do that. My hair will fall out, I'll be nauseous all the time, and then I'd die anyway."

Once home, in hospice care, while filling out a hospital survey, my mom told me, "Don't send it until I'm gone, just in case I end up back in the hospital."

You see, Mom had been honest and candid in filling out the survey. The hospital had made a few mistakes in administering her medications, and she indicated that fact on the survey.

After that, one of us kids were always there. My niece, Anna, even stayed overnight to make sure no other errors occurred with my mom's care.

As soon as the hospital learned Mom had turned down chemo and radiation, they discharged her, and within two hours, we were on our way home. I had to get there to meet the hospice workers and help prepare the house for her homecoming.

In the survey's comments section, Mom wrote, "At least they didn't let the door hit me in the ass once I refused chemo and radiation. It's obviously all about the money!"

Rhoda Kennedy was totally aware of everything happening around her until the last day of her life. We had conversations until that very last day. My mom taught me not to fear death, and she taught me how to die with dignity.

I love you, Mom, and I miss you every day.

Rhoda-Jane is my grandniece. She was diagnosed with B-cell acute lymphocytic leukemia—a blood cancer—at the age of 14 months. Coincidentally, the diagnosis was made on my mom's—Rhoda-Jane's great grandmother's—birthday.

The bone marrow transplant, which was performed six months after the diagnosis, kept Rhoda-Jane in quarantine at Memorial Sloan Kettering Cancer Center for 75 days.

Someday, when she's old enough to understand, we'll tell Rhoda-Jane how brave she was.

At this book printing, Rhoda-Jane is two-and-a-half years old, the cancer is in remission, and she's so happy to be home.

I love her and pray for her every day. I'm positive Rhoda-Jane has guardian angels watching over her, guiding her toward her cure.

Foreword

I am excited and honored that Paula asked me to write the foreword to this book. As I read the passages, I felt reminiscent about the journey I took with Paula and Jack during their struggles towards recovery: medically, in terms of her cancer and, emotionally, through the ups and downs. Many months of frustration and self-doubt, helplessness and hopefulness were shared. Hundreds of hours of prayers from family and friends, including the staff at the Institute for Complementary & Alternative Medicine ICAM and many of our patients, were major parts of Paula's experience and healing.

Paula's story, not boastingly, depicts her strength and courage and is an inspiration for those feeling hopeless, lost and alone when dealing with chronic and life-threatening illness, which was the impetus for her writing this book in the first place.

Guided Cure not only provides the reader with hope and encouragement and instills personal fortitude -it also serves as a valuable source of information on how to find "alternatives" and what questions to ask your healthcare providers. It also "between the lines" exposes deficiencies in mainstream medicine with regards to diagnosing, treatment options and empathy.

The bottom line: Is the hope and expectation that readers will experience *Guided Cure* as an inspiration and a motivation to become aware of their alternatives and to know how to find them. And even though there's a significant difference between information and knowledge and education, *you* are your own best healthcare provider. That said, become an informed consumer of your own healthcare, and take a major role in your healthcare options and decisions. Ask questions and demand answers, second opinions and third opinions. A healthcare provider who dismisses a certain therapy or innovative idea they know nothing about is probably not the right provider for you. There's nothing wrong when your doctor doesn't know, but there's everything wrong when your doctor doesn't listen.

Acknowledge that, without open minds, dreams, passion and compassion, we as a human race would not be where we are in terms of technology and advancement. For instance, there would be no future for us as space explorers because we would be stuck in the Stone Age. Despite the obvious faults, dangers and adversities we've experienced from many of the modern technological advancements, we're now living longer and (I think) better than did our ancestors of just a century ago.

Lastly, complementary-and-alternative-medicine CAM therapies are not only for the ill but the healthy as well. Prevention is key and the absence of symptoms in no way implies the absence of disease. Health is not the *absence* of something- (in this case, illness), but rather the *presence* of an optimized and balanced chemical milieu within the body. So remember: If You Ignore Your Health, It *Will* Leave You!

Yours in Health,

Mark James Bartiss, MD

Chapter 1   Derailed

Can this be happening? It's a few days before Christmas and I'm sitting in the hospital café waiting for my 2:30 appointment with Dr. Stevens. The appointment is to plan my radiation and chemotherapy schedule for the new year. The goal is to dissolve the tumor by February 14.

I can do this. The target date is Valentine's Day. Love can move mountains, right?

I hope so, because I'm scared to death.

The past 30 days have been a blur. I go to the doctor for what I think is a persistent hemorrhoid. But he's not calling it a hemorrhoid. He calls it a mass.

I get a little nervous when he asks another doctor in to confirm what he suspects.

He's not talking to *me* anymore; he's talking to my husband, Jack, saying stuff like "If this was my wife, I would be acting very quickly" and "This is nothing to fool around with."

He immediately orders a colonoscopy. OK, you've got my attention, but please talk to *me*. It's *my* body!

Jack and I have no idea that this is the beginning of what will become a life-changing experience.

We act quickly. Three days later, I have a colonoscopy. A polyp is removed and a biopsy is performed on the mass.

Oh, my God, what a relief.

No cancer!

The doctor still wants the mass removed. So the following week, excision surgery is scheduled.

A done deal. Caught it in time. Merry Christmas! Go on with my happy life.

I have been lucky my whole life. The last time I was in a hospital was 27 years ago, when I gave birth to my daughter Katie.

But this hospital visit is a completely different situation: for surgery, there's a prep the night before — similar to a colonoscopy prep.

I have to be at the hospital early because I'm scheduled to be Dr. Daugherty's second surgery this morning. I chose Dr. Daugherty because of his reputation as one of the best in his field in the tri-state area. Patients travel far distances for his services. I feel confident I'm in good hands.

The registration process is stressful for me because I'm a scaredy-cat when it comes to needles, and I know the IV is coming.

Jack is asked to go to the waiting area.

I'm alone with my thoughts and fears.

All of the hospital staff are professional and courteous. They're cognizant of the fears that overwhelm patients.

I say, "Please don't let me see anything — and get the smelling salts ready."

But things move along much more smoothly than I thought they would. The nursing staff is treating me as if I'm merely getting a spa treatment, keeping me warm with heated blankets.

Once the IV is in place, I'm wheeled down the hall, through double doors, to another area of the building.

I calmly observe all the activity going on. Around what seems to be the command post, different doctors are constantly coming in to consult with anesthesiologists.

The patient next to me answers all the questions she is asked: "What's your name? What are you here for? Who is your doctor?"

She signs the consent forms, and off she goes to the operating room.

It's a busy place. Every few minutes, new patients are brought in and processed. I have a consult with a doctor of anesthesiology, who tells me exactly what's going to happen: "You will be out for only a short amount of time. It's my job to make sure you're comfortable."

As I lie all bundled up in a sort of holding station, more patients come in, their paperwork gets processed at the command post and off they go to surgery.

At one point, the hustle-bustle stops and I'm the only one left. I listen as staff talk about everyday stuff like what they'd watched on TV last night, who they want to win *Dancing with the Stars* and who's their favorite contestant on *The Voice*.

I even hear two doctors passing through, talking about a business opportunity.

Hey, I want in.

Off on the sideline I hear someone say, "Dr. Daugherty's first surgery is having complications."

Uh-oh, it's a good thing I doused myself with lavender, because I don't want my calmness to leave me.

Because I'm the only one left, they let Jack come to stay with me until it's time for surgery.

Thank God I'm comfortable, because this so-called quick procedure is turning into a five-hour ordeal.

I don't know how anyone could recognize me with the hospital garb on, cap and all, but if you keep Jack and me in one place long enough, we're bound to bump into someone we know.

One of our daughter's closest friends who's a nurse is passing through and does a double take.

"Hi, Mrs. B," she calls out.

Recognizing the assisting nurse, she tells us, "It's your lucky day," gently touching the nurse's arm, "This is Marie. She was my mentor when I was training to be a surgical nurse. You're in good hands."

Again, I'm feeling very confident that I'm in the right place at the right time.

Finally, I see Dr. Daugherty at the command post.

They make sure all the paperwork is in order and ask, "What's your name? Who's your doctor? What are you here for?"

Off I go on the gurney, with the nurse, the anesthesiologist, the doctor and a whole crew of assistants surrounding me.

As we go down the hallway, I see one of the nurses inject something into the IV. I question everything, "What is that?"

"That's just in case there's a bug around; this will stop it from getting anywhere near you," she replies.

Good, protect me from any bacteria that may be lurking around, like MRSA.

The operating room is small, full of equipment and very, very bright. I mean Hollywood bright! Lights-camera-action bright.

I look to the left as the anesthesiologist tells me what he's doing. A second later, I'm out.

When I first wake up, while still in a fog, my eyes flutter open and I can see Dr. Daugherty doing paperwork at a desk.

I'm hungry, thirsty and relieved. I'm so happy this is over.

The nurse brings me crackers and juice.

Dr. Daugherty comes over and explains: "I don't like how the tumor looks. Instead of excising the tumor, I decided to first do more biopsies and an ultrasound. It looks like the tumor is in the wall of your colon."

Needless to say, I'm now very *un*happy because the tumor is still there and *they're now calling the mass a tumor!*

Jack can see the disappointment on my face, but he reminds me of the visit I had the night before from the mother of one of my high school friends. She's visiting from Louisiana and came to see us.

Knowing I'm about to have a procedure, she asks, "Can we pray together?"

We all hold hands, and she says the most beautiful prayer: "Lord, we trust in your will. Please keep Paula calm tomorrow. Lord, we know You will send only healing hands to surround her during surgery. Let no harm come to her. We believe You will do what's right for Paula. All our love and trust are in You. Amen."

But now we have to wait a couple of days for the results.

I really want this over with. It's less than two weeks until Christmas, and I still have a lot to do.

At the time, I didn't realize that not cutting into the tumor may have been a godsend.

Three days later, Dr. Daugherty leaves a voice message: "Please, call the office about the biopsy results."

Anxiously, we call back, but every time we try, the office is either closed or we get an answering machine or an answering service. No call back.

After six days, we're pleading with the answering service, "Can we have a courtesy call back, please."

I know the holidays are upon us and everyone's busy, but, come on!

Still no call back.

We figure, no news is good news, right?

Wrong.

I will never forget the feeling. Simply writing about it makes my body composure change and my heart race.

It was one of those defining moments in life: It's 9:30 Monday morning. Jack has a business appointment about 40 minutes away from home. I'm happily puttering around the house.

Phone rings and the caller ID says it's Dr. Daugherty.

I'm glad. Let's get this call over with.

But let me tell you: he definitely catches me off guard by bluntly saying, "You have colorectal cancer."

Period.

"You'll have to start chemotherapy and radiation ASAP."
Period.

"After the tumor shrinks, come back to me. And my only recommendation is a permanent colostomy bag."
Period.

Whoa –! What? Wait a minute. I'm in shock *but* immediately start to ask questions. "What size is the tumor? How fast are the cells growing?"

But he stops my questioning by referring me to the radiology oncologist and medical oncologist he works with at the local hospital.

"They will give you a 'window' of understanding. I'm sorry, but I'm really busy and I have to go."

Ouch! Are you kidding me? I'm starting a living nightmare here.

I sit alone on the family-room couch and cry. Loud cries. I-can't-believe-this-is-happening-to-me cries.

Jack is so far away I can't tell him such news over the phone.

I call my sister, and through my tears, she hears the word *cancer.*

The only thing I remember her saying is, "I'll be right there."

Time must be standing still, because she gets here in a nanosecond.

I'm numb.

I can't believe this is happening!

When Jack gets home, he assures me, "We'll do everything it takes to fight this disease and I'll be beside you every step of the way."

Once I calm down, we make an appointment with Dr. Stevens for Thursday, December 22, 2011, three days before Christmas.

We recognize the radiation oncologist, Dr. Stevens, as a speaker we recently met at a networking event Jack and I attended. We found her to be kind and informative. She, in turn, set me up with the medical oncologist, Dr. Rivers.

"Dr. Rivers and I will work together to combine radiation and chemotherapy in order to shrink or completely dissolve the tumor." Dr. Stevens said.

We meet and the doctors describe the possible side effects.

"At this time," they say, "because the tumor has penetrated the colon wall, it's a stage 3 cancer. The PET scan will determine whether it has metastasized, which would make it stage 4. We want to make sure the cancer is localized and hasn't spread to other areas of your body."

Dr. Rivers orders a PET scan for December 30, 2011.

So much for a happy New Year.

Dr. Stevens and Dr. Rivers say, "There's a possibility that the tumor can be completely dissolved with the one-two punch of radiation and chemo."

This is now my prayer: for the tumor to be completely dissolved.

When my mother was diagnosed with lung cancer, she told me, "If I wasn't depressed, I'd be able to beat this cancer."

Well, guess what, Mom? I'm not depressed and I will beat it. I will beat it. Period.

An appointment is set for January 3, 2012, for tattoos and the first radiation treatment. Yes, that's right: I'm going to get tattoos on my heinie.

I won't bore you with the 24-hour pity party I threw myself. I don't have time to cry. I have to wrap my head around the daily radiation and chemo that is scheduled to take place in the new year.

Here's an excerpt from my journal dated 12-22-11: "I already know that I'm blessed to have a strong family support system. Jack has made sure I have a history of excellent nutrition. I am physically fit. I have a deep faith. I know I am being watched over."

As my mother used to say, "Thank you, Jesus."

"Let Operation Dissolve begin!"

Chapter 2   Good Vibrations

I'm unusually calm during the Christmas and New Year holidays. My journal says stuff like "Fun tailgate party at Sunsplash.

We exchanged gifts and holiday spirits!

Christmas Eve. Yoga/work/16 dinner guests.

'Tis the season!

I feel great."

We have a very nice Christmas and a relaxing day after but it's the calm before the storm.

On December 27, we travel 50 miles away to a university hospital to get a second opinion on the surgery, to see Dr. Polanski, who is recommended by the original doctor who found the tumor.

The hospital is very large. *I don't like it.* There are long waiting lines, and the receptionist has the sniffles. No one seems to know what's going on. After 40 minutes, we're told we have to reschedule because Dr. Polanski has been called to perform an emergency surgery.

Please! I got up at 7 a.m. and drove 50 miles. How long could this surgery possibly be? *I had an appointment, for crying out loud.*

The sniffling receptionist says, "I'm sorry but Dr. Polanski has canceled and would like to reschedule."

Well, guess what? That's not happening. Jack and I will go to a different doctor for a second opinion.

Besides, when I visited the bathroom, the soap dispenser was empty. Really? We're in a hospital; no wonder the receptionist has the sniffles.

It's frustrating — definitely not like a day at the spa.

I vent my frustration the whole ride home. I'm so lucky to have Jack with me at all the appointments. He's calm, cool, and collected. Plus, he's reasonable — and, well, I'm not.

I'm mentally preparing myself for a visit with my brother. He's coming over after work tomorrow. I'm sure he's wondering why I want to see him. It's unusual for me to ask him to come over instead of just talking by phone.

He's an attorney, so he probably thinks I need legal advice.

I waited until after the Christmas holidays, because my news is so unpleasant. It's the kind of news that has to sink in—information you just don't give over the phone.

I'm uneasy as I wait for my brother to arrive. I greet him at the door, we exchange pleasantries, I offer him a drink and we sit at the kitchen table.

He asks, "OK, so what's up?"

Without hesitation, like ripping off a Band-Aid, I blurted out, "There's no easy way to say this. I have cancer."

I can tell this is the last thing he thought I was going to tell him. His facial expression exhibits sadness; I can almost see his heart sink. He has no words. He gets up from his seat, comes over to me and, with tears in his eyes, hugs me.

It was indeed hard to say it aloud. We cry, we hug and we talk about how I'm going to beat this cancer.

It's hard to tell people. The hardest person to tell is my daughter, Katie. Both of us blocked it out. Neither one of us can remember much. I remember only the feeling. You never want to hurt your child and I know this is going to devastate her. Her first thought is, *Oh, my God, my mother is going to die.*

I've decided to tell people only if absolutely necessary. I told my brother and I then tell my sisters, just in case something happens during the treatments. I have no idea how the chemo and radiation are going to affect me. I tell key friends who I know will be supportive and stay positive. I don't want any negative cancer vibes around me.

Right now, not many people know about it and I like it that way. I can enjoy myself without people thinking, "Why is she having so much fun when she has cancer?"

People say things they would never say if they knew I had cancer. I don't want people to think they have to be careful about what they say in front of me.

The worst is when they *do* know and you get that puppy dog look of pity that I can't stand. People just don't know what to say.

It's hard for me to believe, but I find out that two of my high school girlfriends and one friend of 25 years have experienced cancer firsthand in the past few years.

The way I found out about one of them is one of the reasons I want to keep my own cancer news to myself.

I was at ShopRite and I bumped into someone I haven't seen in a long time. We catch up on local news in the bakery section.

She lowered her voice and said "You did hear about So-and-So, right?"

I'm curious, so I replied, "No, what?"

"She has [lowered her voice a little bit more, almost to a whisper] cancer!"

When people learn someone has cancer, there's apparently some unknown reason they just have to tell someone what they heard. I was calling that kind of talk *cancer gossip* way before cancer happened to me and I don't want to be part of someone's cancer gossip.

I feel strongly about someone else's negative cancer thoughts coming my way. There's research out there about thoughts having energy.

I want to surround myself only with people who believe I can beat this. Besides, it's absolutely exhausting telling people about it.

Tomorrow is the PET scan. Knowing I'd be anxious, I arrange for Jack and me to get massages today. The massage is wonderful. Both of us need one so much. Then I treat myself to a mani/pedi. Relax . . . Relax . . ..

I make it through the PET scan with a little help from Xanax. They put radioactive glucose into my veins, and now I have to wait forty-five minutes for the substance to circulate throughout my body. After the wait, they take X-rays. Cancer loves sugar, so the glucose will go directly where the cancer is. I have to stay still for twenty-five minutes during the scan. They take extra pictures of my pelvic area. I'm glad it's over. The tube that encircles me is confining.

We have a relaxing New Year's Eve at home, exactly where I want to be. My sister, Susan, comes over for dinner. She put Rogers and Hammerstein's song "Impossible" from the Disney story *Cinderella* on my cell phone as a ring tone. *So much fun.* Every time she calls, I hear "Impossible things are happening every day."
I've placed positive affirmations where I can easily see them daily. I'm doing everything in my power to stay positive.
I imagine the tumor gone.
Plop plop, fizz fizz. Gone.
I expect good things to happen.

It's January 2. I try to relax because I start radiation and chemo tomorrow. I do a one-hour yoga class and come home to an Epsom salt bath. I run the hot water and slip out of my housecoat. The water is just the right temperature.

I just read that orange essential oil is good against cancer, so I decide to put some in the bath. I start adding a few drops. It smells so good that I add ten more drops and start lifting the water and splashing it all over myself.

Well, in less than a minute, I experience a sudden allergic reaction, and my legs and my bottom get hives like red blotches all over them. *So, not relaxing.*

Without my knowledge, to set the mood, Jack had lit a candle, but in my frenzy I unwittingly throw my housecoat over it and almost start a fire.

My phone starts to ring.

"Impossible things are happening every day" starts playing.

It's Susan.

With a computer at her fingertips, she had googled *essential oils and Epsom salt* and found you can mix Epsom salt with all oils except—you guessed it: citrus oils.

I know these oils are powerful. You really have to know what you're doing when mixing them. Apparently, it's a well-known fact that you shouldn't mix salt and citrus.

It takes about thirty minutes for the irritation to subside.

I'm glad this happened before the start of radiation, because I definitely would have concluded that the radiation had had something to do with that rash reaction.

Chapter 3   Radiation

Stacy and Deena are my radiation technicians. I really like them, which is good because I'll see them every weekday for the next six weeks. I'm very happy that my standing appointment is at 10 a.m. the first appointment of the day. In and out within an hour.

A mold is made of my torso and thighs to pinpoint the radiation and to keep me in the same position for each treatment. I lie on the table, facedown. Once I'm in position, a circular machine surrounds the table. I have to stay motionless in the machine for twenty minutes while the radiation targets the tumor.

The first treatment is a learning experience because you don't know what's going to happen. *I'm clueless.*

The radiation looks like a beam of light. The beam of light lines up with the tattoos on my hip area which, in turn, lines up with the tumor, so that the tumor gets targeted with the radiation. Many beams are coming from all different directions. Once the techs make sure I'm positioned correctly on the table, they leave the room to stand behind a protective wall that has a small window so they can watch me. I can hear their voices on what sounds like a microphone that projects into the room from the other side of the wall.

"Are you comfortable?"

I lie there rigid on the table, "Yes, as comfortable as I'm going to get."

"OK, I'm going to walk you through this. The table is going to move a couple times during the treatment. Everything is going to be all right, and you're going to be fine. Try to relax."

First my heart starts to pound and every minute seems like an hour.

After a few minutes, they check on me: "How are you doing?" comes over the microphone.

"I'm fine." Which is not true, for now my mouth is completely dry and terror has set in. Nothing is hurting, though, except for my thoughts. I was thinking, *this radiation must be harmful because they're going behind a steel wall so that none of the radiation can get anywhere near them.*

It is so quiet I can hear only the machine's mechanical noises caused by the moving around. *It's going to be a long six weeks.*

By the third treatment, I'm filled with anxiety.

I feel claustrophobic.

I visualize taking a walk around Eagle Lake to soothe my angst. Eagle Lake is a Pocono Mountains resort Jack and I have enjoyed for many years.

It takes about 45 minutes to walk around the lake. *In my mind's eye, I'm walking around the lake. I stop at the water fall and then at the marina.* Thinking about it helps a little.

Somehow I get around the lake in ten minutes, instead of forty-five. *I look at all the pretty wildflowers on the berm. The sun is glistening on the lake water and there's one lone boat with two fishermen in it, directly in the middle of the lake.* The machine starts to move and my thoughts completely vanish.

I have to work on my meditation skills. Even though the treatment's a daily occurrence, it's not getting any easier.

It's week two of radiation and Stacy and Deena play soothing, meditative music, while I get my treatment today. The music definitely helps lower my anxiety levels.

Once a week, Jack and I meet with the doctor. Dr. Stevens is on vacation, so we see Dr. Silverberg today. Jack and Dr. Silverberg knew each other from being in the One & Done club in the '70s at Greco's Bar, which was in the Burg, also known as Chambersburg, in Trenton. The purpose of the One & Done club is to have only one drink, after which you're done and you have to go home. That rarely happened.

I can't go anywhere without Jack's knowing someone. But Jack's popularity is not helping with my wanting to keep the cancer diagnosis to myself. He even knew the janitor we bumped into on the hospital elevator today.

Everything is going well. So far, the only thing getting the best of me is the anxiety. Sometimes I feel pressure back there. At night, I pass bloody mucusy stuff. I think it's the tumor. Really. It looks just like it. The doctor calls it chaffing.

They keep asking me about my pain levels, which is scary because I don't have any pain right now.

It's Friday the 13th. Fourteen days of radiation treatments down, and four weeks to go. I'll finish radiation on February 14.

Double treatment has started. I call it Operation Dissolve and Delete. When you delete the messages on your phone, the messages jump right into the garbage can. I visualize the cancer going into the garbage.

I say to myself, "The chemo will delete the cancer."

I also have a picture of Pac-Man on the front of my phone to remind me that the cancer will have dissolved by the end of radiation.

You get to know the people in the waiting room. The room is small. There's seating for eight people. A set of four lockers are in one corner, and a TV hangs from the ceiling in another corner. Conveniently, there's a bathroom attached so you can change into your hospital gown.

Sarah and Rob are the appointment after me. Rob has esophageal cancer and trouble swallowing. We pray for each other. Rob, Sarah and Jack get great dinner ideas by watching Rachael Ray's TV show, while I get my treatment.

Lorna has breast cancer. She comes in with her sister daily. It's scary enough to have to go through this, but Lorna scares me even more every day by saying, "Girl, you are gonna to be all burnt up by the end of radiation."

She always comes late and causes a ruckus. I look forward to the end of her treatments. Cancer doesn't discriminate, everyone in the waiting room has a different type, and we're all in different age-groups.

I know I've said it before and I'll say it again: I love this hospital!

Today Stacy asks, "How were you feeling last night?"

"Pretty good, I had a relaxing evening."

"I was thinking about you last night and wrapped my arms around you and hoped you felt it," she says.

Wow, I'm not just a cancer patient here: I'm a person who feels loved. I feel safe here. This radiation team of Dr. Stevens, Stacy and Deena are going to dissolve and delete the cancer in six weeks.

That's the goal.

No surgery will be needed.

It's been more than a week since the PET scan. It's hard waiting for results. I can't say no news is good news. That didn't work for me with the last biopsy. Either way, I'm confident that the chemo and radiation will kill all the cancer.

Jack had to call the emergency number to get information about the PET scan and the chemo drugs. Great news: no cancer has spread. It's a stage 3 cancer. Because it's localized, I start on chemo pills tomorrow. A thousand milligrams in the morning and a thousand milligrams at night. I'm feeling good. I'm ready to kick some cancer butt—no pun intended.

Jack and I are turning into an old married couple. We're having a lively debate over the exact time I should take the Xeloda. One paper says thirty minutes *after* a meal and one says *within* thirty minutes after finishing a meal. This is crazy. Jack wants me to take it *exactly* thirty minutes after a meal, and I think it would be OK *between* twenty and thirty minutes after a meal. So silly. "Marital bliss."

Xango juice was introduced to me several years ago by a networking friend who had back pain. Jack himself deals with arthritis pain, so we try the juice and, in a short amount of time, Jack's arthritis pain disappears. I'm so impressed with the result that we do a little research on the juice and learn it has been used by traditional healers for centuries.

Found primarily in Southeast Asia is a fruit called mangosteen, which is the main ingredient in Xango juice. Mangosteen is nature's greatest source of xanthones, which are just as impressive as they sound: they're phytonutrients with powerful anti-inflammatory properties that help boost the immune system.

So, we each added two ounces of Xango juice three times a day to our daily supplement routines.

At a health summit, shortly after our discovery of the juice, I hear a woman who lives in Ewing, New Jersey — not far from where I live — tell her story about dealing with a second bout of breast cancer. First time around the chemo and radiation had knocked her out, leaving her with low to no energy.

Second time around, she says, she decided to do the twenty-one-day Xango juice challenge, which consists of drinking an entire bottle of Xango — 750 milliliters — and a gallon of distilled water daily for twenty-one days. She says that by her second set of chemo treatments she was able to attend the theater and go out dancing in New York. She didn't miss a single event in her life the second time around.

She gave all the credit to Xango.

Little did I know that within a few years, I would be considering the twenty-one-day Xango challenge for myself. I'm such a lucky lady: Once I made the request to the local Xango community, thirty bottles got donated and showed up at my doorstep. I will drink a full bottle of Xango with a gallon of distilled water every day during the chemo and radiation treatments.

I feel sure the tumor in my body will be gone in six weeks.

Chapter 4   The Kennedy Women Talk

Susan is coming over for dinner and to color my hair. If laughter is good for cancer, Susan is the cure. She soon has me laughing about many things, such as politics, the way British people talk and the licorice candy Good & Plenty.

She's singing, "Charlie says, 'Love my Good & Plenty.' Charlie says, 'It really rings the bell.' Charlie says, 'Love my Good & Plenty. Don't know any other candy that I love so well.'" You name it, and Susan can talk and laugh about it.

My sister Lois leaves goodies in my "magic metal milk box" on the front porch. When I get home today, there's frankincense and myrrh body spray and orange and lavender mist—all of the scents good for curing cancer— and a yoga water bottle. I'm going to smell really good in yoga class. I love my sisters.

My mother's maiden name is Kennedy.

Mom loved her Irish heritage, and she always said, "Kennedy woman are strong women."

She would say, "My grandmother Margaret Brennan married James Thaddeus Collins. They were Irish immigrants and came to the United States of America for opportunities. They left Ireland because of the Great Famine and for a better life."

As young kids, my sisters and I loved listening to family stories. Especially when all of the aunts and uncles were sitting around the dining room table after a holiday dinner.

"Your great grandmother was a strong women who endured intolerable conditions as a steerage passenger on a two to three-month trip from Ireland to Ellis Island."

"She was sponsored into the United States by Mary and Michael Gorman. They were affectionately called Mom and Pop Gorman."

"Once in Brooklyn, Margaret and James Thaddeus had a baby girl, Anna Mary Collins, your Grandmom."

"When Grandmom was seven months old her mother died at only twenty-four years old." *That part of the story always made me sad.*

"Back then, in 1894, men were not thought to be capable of raising an infant. Therefore, the Gorman's—who were from the same village in Ireland that Grandmom's mother came from and who also sponsored her in this country—raised Anna Mary as their own daughter, along with their natural daughter, Esther Agatha, as Anna Mary's sister. When Esther got older, everyone referred to her as Old Aunt Essie."

It was an informal adoption.

Anna Mary married James Joseph Kennedy in 1915 and had seven kids: Jimmy, Gerard, Essie, Betty, Lawrence, Anne and Eileen Rhoda.

"Dancing Jim, as they called him, made Grandmom a Kennedy woman."

"Your grandmother became a widow at the age of forty-one. She had to raise seven children, ages three to nineteen years old, alone."

"First she lost her husband. Then she suffered the loss of a three-year old toddler; and later, an adult son. Baby Anne was born between me and Uncle Lawrence. She had a cardiac condition that would be corrected easily today. I often wonder what it would have been like to have a sister close in age."

"My brother, James Joseph II, Anna Mary's first born, died at the early age of 35 from cancer. He served in World War II in a hazardous waste-disposal unit. Probably the cause of the cancer."

My mother always told me, "It doesn't matter what happens in your life. You are a survivor. You can handle any of life's storms. Always remember that you're a Kennedy woman. And Kennedy women are strong."

I want Katie to know: You are exactly what I asked for. I wanted a baby girl. I got one. I wanted a strong, independent woman. You turned into one.

And when I complained during your teenage years, your grandma would remind me, "Katie is exactly what you ordered."

I want Katie to know how strong she is. When life gets tough, we Kennedy women have a deep well within us that we can draw from. An inner strength. My inner strength is my faith. I know that Katie, too, has that faith. I want Katie to know how proud I am of the woman she has become. Soooo, no time like the present.

I call Katie while Jack and I are driving to the hospital for a radiation treatment, "Hi, Katie, I have to tell you something."

Katie says, "Ma, I worked late last night, and you just woke me up.

I can't help laughing. "You've got to love me Kate."

We have the "Kennedy women" talk. It's now on Katie's tapes. My mother also repeated herself over and over again.

If we said, "Mom, you said that four times already," she would say, "I know, but I want to make sure it gets on your tapes." As if each of us had a little recorder in our heads. Well, it worked. I still hear my mother's voice in my head. And now I'm doing the same thing to Katie.

Chapter 5   Surgery?

My friends, Tom and Patti, own a jewelry store and they ask me to work the store while they vacation in Florida for a couple weeks.

Knowing I'd try anything to rid myself of the cancer, when they return, they give me healing crystals.

Tom says, "I carefully picked out each crystal. Adventurine is the green one. It's a quartz that settles nausea and dissolves negative thoughts."

"Chrysocolla is good for meditation and great for invoking inner strength and joy," Patti continues. "We picked amethyst because it's a positive stone that removes negative energy. It has protective elements and a high spiritual vibration that will help you stay focused."

Tom and Patti remind me a lot of me and Jack, - especially when it comes to marital competition.

For instance, when he thinks Patti isn't listening, Tom says, "I picked out the best and most powerful stones." Holding out a crystal in his hand he says, "This one is a Tibetan quartz which is the most powerful healing and energy amplifier on the planet. I found this one."

"No you don't," Patti chimes in. "I always find better *stones* than you. Besides they're called *crystals*, not *stones*. I found the rose quartz and it's by far the best because it's the crystal of unconditional love and infinite peace. It brings deep inner healing and self-love."

I interrupt their bickering, "Hey, tell me more about your vacation."

Patti starts to tell a story. "We did have one incident by the pool on our second-to-last day."

Tom rolls his eyes.

"I'm floating in the pool with a cocktail, and I start to wonder where Tom is," she says. "All of a sudden, I see him walking towards the pool, looking annoyed and disturbed, and he has two hotel security guards – on either side of him.

Instead of being worried about *him*, I immediately accuse: "What did *you* do?'"

Tom takes over, "Yeah, Patti thinks *I* did something wrong, when all it was was that I'd gotten stuck in the men's bathroom for a half hour.

At first, I think it's kind of funny.

But when the door doesn't budge, I start to bang on it.

No one hears me, and, I bang harder.

Now it's not funny anymore.

Panic sets in."

Patti smirks, but Tom continues to tell the story.

"My hands start to bleed I'm banging so hard.

I start to sweat and now I'm getting freaked out.

I take the toilet paper holder apart with hopes there's something I can use to pry open the door."

Patti giggles. "All the while I'm relaxing in the pool."

Tom continues. "Finally, someone hears my banging and calls security. I'm extremely happy to hear my rescuers on the other side of the door. In order to free me, they have to take the door completely off by removing the hinges.

Still smiling Patti adds, "Yeah, I'm married to MacGyver. At least we got a comped night out of the ordeal."

"I would rather have had a normal dinner at one of the restaurants," Tom mumbles.

"At check-out, all of the desk clerks were staring and pointing at Tom because he was the talk of the morning report. They called it the 'bathroom incident.'"

My friends made it home safely from vacation, and I love my crystals.

Never a dull moment with Patti and Tom. They also keep me busy. They take me to Rotary Club lunches. We attend fundraising events, like the New Hope, Pennsylvania's Fire & Ice Ball and take trips to Atlantic City for a weekend.

I always tell them, "You guys are like Energizer bunnies."

Massage therapists and other natural healers frequently visit the jewelry store looking for specific crystals. These healers swear by the crystal's power.

To this day, either the crystals are with me in my pocketbook or they're on top of the TV in the family room.

I left them out all night the last full moon so they can reenergize.

I will leave no stone unturned.

Pun intended.

For gentle yoga, meditation or just plain fun, I go to the gym almost every day. Weekends are busy with breakfast with the girls, non-profit City of Angels NJ open house, and the HOB chili cook-off.

Jack's going to win the chili contest this year.

I'm staying very positive. As long as I'm busy, it keeps my mind from cancer thoughts.

Miracles happen.

I believe in the power of prayer.

My prayer warriors are working overtime.

And I believe in angels, too.

We make an appointment with Dr. Sylvia Patel at another university hospital in Philadelphia. Dr. Patel is a colon and rectal specialist who has won awards every year since 2001. I'm lucky to get an appointment with her so quickly for a second opinion.

Today is Monday, January 23, 2012, and it's review time with Dr. Stevens, who says, "Keep your eye on the prize, and the prize is: your life."

We talk about the possibility of surgery.

Dr. Stevens had a meeting with Dr. Daugherty, the surgeon. "Still, Dr. Daugherty's only option for you is a permanent stoma," she says.

Stoma is the term for colostomy.

"Even if the tumor is completely gone?"

"Yes, that's his recommendation," she says.

"That's a red flag for me. Why would I have a life-changing surgery if the tumor is gone?"

Dr. Stevens highly recommends a second opinion — which I have already scheduled for February 6 with Dr. Patel.

"Surgery should take place within six weeks from the end of radiation and chemo. Otherwise, scar tissue will form, making it a more difficult surgery."

Harder for whom?

So, I ask, "What if I don't have surgery? What if I wait to see whether the cancer comes back and if it does, then do the surgery?"

I'll have to clarify this, but my interpretation of the answer is, my only choice will be chemo.

"You have only one shot with radiation because of the scar tissue that forms."

I think about Patti's story of Tom getting stuck in the bathroom. To free him they had to remove the hinges to open the door.

I feel unhinged; I need an open door to new opportunities. Please God, help me, guide me.

It's the end of January and the weeks are flying by.

My sister, Lois, calls to say, "I got you an appointment with my holistic doctor for 2:15 p.m. on Presidents' Day."

Before I could object about the cost, Lois says: "And it's my treat. That's how important it is to me that you meet him."

"That's the day before Jack's birthday."

"Then that's my gift to you *and* Jack."

The doctor is willing to see me this quickly as a favor to Lois because she's been his patient for years.

He's located in Manahawkin near Long Beach Island, New Jersey, and he's coming in on a day the office is supposed to be closed.

If you ever want to help a person who has a cancer diagnosis, give the person cash. Time off from work, the cost of gas for traveling to and from doctors' visits, parking fees, and many other unexpected expenses can put a burden on a family's finances.

Tick tock, tick tock, four weeks down, two more weeks of radiation left. My rear end is sore, and it burns when I pee.

I can handle this.

I will be cancer free soon.

No surgery for me.

It's Monday, February 1, and Dr. Stevens is treating me as an individual, not a protocol. She keeps telling me: "Keep your eye on the prize. You don't know which percentage you will be. Your *first* shot at killing cancer is your *best* shot. Cancer is unpredictable, because the guy you think won't make it lasts ten more years, and the one with the best chance can die in a year."

"You'll make the right decision when the time comes. One day at a time."

The radiology techs still treat me as if the tumor will be gone by the end of the treatments.

I feel like it's gone already. Really. The pressure is gone even if my heinie hurts from the radiation, like bad sunburn in my private areas.

I can handle this, as long as it's gone by the end of February.

It's possible that next Monday, when Dr. Patel does the scope, she'll tell me there's nothing there.

Impossible, things are happening every day.

This Thursday I give Deena, the radiology technician, some peppermint oil to try.

She's looking for a little extra energy and peppermint is supposed to give a boost.

On Friday, she asks for more peppermint.

"I love it," she says. "Yesterday the oil kept me going all day."

So Stacy, the other tech says, "Let me try some."

She slathers it on her temples.

Come Monday, I put some peppermint oil on myself to help ease nausea. I go into the treatment room and Stacy says, "I can't take that peppermint oil."

I think it's because I had just put some on. *Well, oh my goodness:* Stacy lifts up her blonde hair, and it looks as if something has scorched her temples.

She tells me, "It got worse every day and the blotches moved around my face all weekend long."

Now, I have the entire radiology department talking about the patient who almost sent one of the technicians to the emergency room.

I call the girl I get the oils from and she says, "There has to be something out of balance in the technician's body for the oil to have caused such a harsh reaction. People who know they have sensitive skin should always test a small area before using the oils freely."

Every Monday, Jane takes my vitals before I see the doctor. This Monday, she starts to ask questions like, "Paula, what kind of vitamins are you taking? And, "How about herbs: are you taking any herbs?"

"No, nothing."

Jane says, "Really? I've heard about your oils!"

Jack has been right a lot lately. You really need someone with you when you're talking to the doctor. He's right about using Preparation H with steroids. You can use steroids but not lavender oil. Go figure.

Jack's also right about the number of treatments left and about not putting ointment on the burned area until after the treatments.

"Radiation will intensify the area the ointment is placed on."

Dr. Stevens says, "You must drive Jack crazy."

I say, "I have Jack believing he's the luckiest guy in Hamilton Square, maybe even in all of New Jersey."

The truth is, I'm the lucky one!

Chapter 6　　　　　Second Opinion

It's Friday and my last radiation treatment of the week. Only one more week of radiation left. Today I have a scan to tighten the margins. This will help the last five treatments to concentrate directly on the tumor area, even if the tumor is gone! They call it a *boost*.

It's Monday, and we're at the University of Pennsylvania to get a second opinion on the surgery. Dr. Sylvia Patel is gentle, kind and compassionate, but her words still sting. She answers all of my questions.

Bottom line is, "If you choose not to operate, there is an 85 percent chance the cancer will come back."

When I ask, "Why can't I wait and, if the cancer comes back, then operate?"

She replies, "If the cancer comes back, your chances of survival will be 20 percent.

The tumor is still there.

And because of its location, the only surgical option is a permanent colostomy."

She was acquainted with – and touted – Dr. Daugherty: "He, in my opinion, is the best colorectal surgeon in New Jersey."

I feel devastated. I was so hopeful that after all the radiation and four weeks of chemo, this doctor was going to tell me the tumor was gone.

This is the first time I feel defeated.

Back in radiation oncology, Dr. Stevens is trying to help me wrap my head around the surgery. The reality of it has not sunk in. They gave me booklets about colostomies; they gave me information on support groups. None of it is working. My brain is not accepting that I'll be living my life very differently in a few months. It's just not registering. I won't do it!

As we're leaving Dr. Stevens's office, Dr. Polanski, from the first university hospital, calls my cell phone to reschedule the appointment he missed. I take the call on a bench in the lobby of the hospital.

Jack and I each have one ear leaning into the phone as we listen to Dr. Polanski quoting the same statistics as the other doctors did: "There is an 85 percent chance that the cancer will come back if we don't operate."

He, too, praises Dr. Daugherty, but adds: "I will do the surgery laparoscopically. The selling point is a smaller incision, which means a shorter recovery time."

I put my hand over the phone and Jack read my lips: "I do not want surgery."

I am completely overwhelmed.

As suggested, I meet with a girl who had had the surgery many years ago. Her three-year-old son and one of his friends are running around the kitchen table, thereby keeping her young.

"As you can see, my life is very normal. You, too, will get used to it." She smiles as she picks up crayons scattered all over the kitchen floor.

Then, pointing at her stomach, she says, "You just have to keep it clean to avoid infection."

I'm still not buying it. *I can't accept this.*

What I *can* accept is my body's healing itself. That is what I believe. I believe that if you build up and strengthen your immune system your body can and will heal itself. I'd like to at least give it a try.

But fear is a funny thing. My heart, my soul and my gut tell me *not* to have this surgery. But my logic, based on the fear put into my mind by the doctors, leads me to believe that maybe I *should* have the surgery.

Oh, my God, I'm so confused. This is a major decision. I have some soul searching to do. Do I do what my gut is telling me to do? Or do I listen to what every single medical professional is telling me I must do to save my life.

It's Friday, February 14, Happy Valentine's Day. It's my last day of radiation treatments. So appropriate that it's Valentine's Day because I truly love this radiation team. Stacy, Deena and Dr. Stevens have set the bar very high with regard to the way patients should be treated. I saw these radiation technicians five days a week for six weeks.

In the beginning, it seemed it would be a long time. Today, I feel as if it flew by. The technicians give me a Hallmark card that says: "There is a circle of caring around you. And you are right in the middle." That is exactly how I feel. They made one of the scariest times in my life bearable. They also wrote beautiful, encouraging words inside the card. If I'm ever having a bad day, I can read this card and regain the confidence I need to carry on.

From Stacy: "We know you'll make it through this. You'll make the best of whatever is thrown at you. You're strong and beautiful and a confident go-getter. For sure, we know you'll always turn those -lemons into lemonade-. Always know there are at least two Earth angels on your side. We love you. Happy Graduation Day!"

From Deena: "You are an extraordinary woman who will find the positive in any situation. I have no doubt that your attitude, drive and determination will cure you. Both Stacy and I have grown by knowing you. You will always be in our hearts. Love, Deena P.S. You can do this. Take that surgery by the balls and own it!" Deena signed it, *Your, asshole buddy.* Deena always knew how to make me laugh. But I still believe I can beat the odds and be in the 15 percent who survive without surgery.

Dr. Stevens's main objective today was to make sure I make doctor's appointments with the surgeon and the medical oncologist, which I did. Next week is doctors week for me: February 20, Dr. Mark Bartiss, an alternative/complementary doctor. February 21, happy birthday Jack, and back to Dr. Stevens to check my progress post-radiation.

I've been taking oxycodone every four hours, even through the night, to get relief. My ass is almost burned off. Every nook and cranny is peeling. And it's very painful. I have to regulate with Dulcolax because the oxycodone causes constipation and very painful BMs. Feels like a baseball, but comes out the size of a pea. Ouch! I know, too much information. Dr. Stevens even let me skip the last couple of treatments. There was no use burning me more, because the plan is to have surgery within the next six weeks.

Last, Dr. Daugherty the surgeon, on February 23 at 3:30 p.m. Back-to-back doctor's appointments.

I'd better get some rest!

Chapter 7   Doctors Week

Dr. Bartiss spends two and a half hours with me, Jack and my sister, Lois. He wants to know everything about me. He spends time on my medical history, but he also wants to know about my childhood. How do I look at life? What is my attitude? Is my glass half empty or half full? He asks a lot of questions. I answer them as best as I can.

I feel defeated. I'm drugged up on oxycodone and, everywhere I go I bring my own cushion to sit on, because I'm so burnt up it's painful to sit.

So far, all the doctors have me believing there will be an operation by the end of March—certainly no later than the second week in April.

Dr. Bartiss talks to me about ozone therapy--through a process called major autohematherapy—and biophotonic therapy—also called ultraviolet blood irradiation (UBI).

He says, "I'll take eight ounces of your blood, treat it with the same volume of a gas called ozone, which is manufactured from 100 percent oxygen and exposed to ultra violet light. Once treated with germicidal light, the blood is returned to the same site it was taken from. The sick cells are targeted and the healthy cells remain intact. This, in essence, creates a self-generated vaccine. OZONE and UBI stimulate the immune system."

"Jack and I are excited about giving my immune system a boost. That's been one of our concerns," I say.

Chemo and radiation wreak havoc on the immune system. Another reason I question the quick surgery.

"Why would they want to operate on someone with a weakened immune system?" I ask.

We talk about possibly getting some treatments in before the medical oncologist orders the PET scan.

Of course, I want to do my own research on this treatment, so Jack and I tell Dr. Bartiss,

"We want to think about it and will get back to you in a couple of days."

We also have to figure out where the money for this alternative treatment is going to come from, because it is not covered by health insurance. All in all, we leave the appointment feeling excited about the possibilities.

February 21. "Happy birthday Jack!" The beginning of the office visit with Dr. Stevens goes well.

First, there's, of course, the obligatory small talk: "How's your family?"

"Fine."

"How was your week?"

"OK, I guess."

"How is your rear end doing?"

"My rear is still really burned and, instead of getting better, it seems to be getting worse."

"Radiation works like a microwave oven: it continues to intensify well after the treatments end."

She offers me some cream samples for my rear. She makes sure I made all the doctor's appointments. Dr. Daugherty's appointment is tomorrow.

"I'm not happy that your appointment with the medical oncologist isn't until March 14."

"That's Dr. Rivers first available appointment," I say.

Dr. Stevens rolls her eyes to show her displeasure.

I'm OK with it, because I want time to slow down. I have a lot of thinking to do.

Dr. Stevens says, "I'm not a fan of laparoscopic surgery. The old-fashioned kind of surgery would be better because the surgeon would be able to see better, it's more thorough and the surgeon can more easily move the organs around."

The visit takes a turn for the worse when I start to ask questions about surgery and why I have to do it so quickly.

I tell the doctor, "I want my body to have a chance to build up its immune system. I want survival percentages."

She says, "Only 15 percent of patients survive without surgery."

Everyone is reading the same book. All the doctors quote the same percentages.

I question, "Why can't I be in the 15 percent who live without having the operation? I don't want the operation. I would do it only because I'm expected to follow doctor's orders."

"We had a conversation a couple of weeks ago, remember? You told me, 'Don't listen to what anyone else says about your healthcare decisions, - not Jack, not your sisters, not your daughter, no one.' You said, 'Listen only to yourself.' Well, I've done that and I don't feel good about having surgery. How current is the research you're quoting me about?"

Dr. Stevens says, "I don't like your attitude. Maybe you should talk to someone about it."

I guess she means a therapist.

Just for the record: I have not skipped anything on my schedule since finding out I have cancer. The people who know I have cancer tell me how proud they are of my attitude. I didn't roll up in a ball and cry, "Why me?"

I've done everything they've asked of me from day one — and quickly.

I'm flipping out on the inside, thinking, *How dare she say that to me?* On the outside, I stay calm, cool and collected. After all, she does have the white coat on — and she just now suggested I needed psychiatric help.

That's red flag number two. Remember, red flag number one was when I was told, "Even if the tumor is gone, we still feel you should have surgery."

I can't overemphasize the fact that someone should be with you when you talk with doctors. You don't want to miss important information. And you don't want to misconstrue what a doctor may be suggesting. Jack, too, senses a change in the atmosphere when I don't jump on the express surgery bandwagon.

The visit is tense and we leave it that I will make another appointment after I see the medical oncologist on March 14.

All the doctors work as a team, so I'm sure they discuss my case weekly. And I'm even more sure they're not happy with me at this point because I'm not agreeing to the surgery.

Of course, I beat this bad-attitude "dead horse" with anyone who will listen. Poor Jack hears it the whole ride home. Later, when I vent again with my sisters, he has to hear it all over again.

Dr. Bartiss calls later in the afternoon to let me know two of his patients may call me to tell me about their treatment experiences. I tell him about my "bad attitude."

Dr. Bartiss says, "Don't burn your bridges, because you may need that surgery."

When I tell him, "Jack and I are excited about starting the treatments you suggested," he says, "I just got goosebumps."

He goes on, "In terms of my medical care, whenever I get goosebumps patients should heed what I'm saying because, thus far, it's ended up being 100 percent spot on!"

He then adds, "The treatments may render you cancer free by the time you get the PET scan."

This is one of those times I feel I'm being watched over from above. The PET scan will probably be in late March or early April, because my appointment with the medical oncologist isn't until mid-March. So, that'll give me time to see whether these alternative treatments make a difference.

Only time will tell.

The first call I get comes from a guy named Frank. After introducing himself, the first thing he says is: "Don't let it get you down. Start acting as if you're already healed."

Frank says he had bladder cancer and that his tumor was the size of an orange.

"I shot ozone five times into my bladder and had three ultraviolet/ozone treatments."

When he went to his conventional doctor for a checkup and biopsy, the doctor was surprised because he couldn't tell where the tumor had been removed. The area where the tumor had been was remarkably cleared up.

"The doctor said, 'I've never seen this kind of positive result in such a short amount of time,'" Frank says.

"He told me, 'Keep up the good work,'" but never asked me what I had been doing."

Frank raves about Dr. Bartiss' treatments. He keeps saying: "The treatments won't hurt you. They can only help you." He talks about extra energy and the mental clarity that he experiences with the treatments.

He says, "My dentist says, 'Ozone sterilizes everything.' Dr. Bartiss strongly recommended that I change my eating habits. I did, and my cholesterol lowered and my prostate numbers got better."

He wishes me well and I thank him for the call.

When Paul calls, he says, "I've had to take Celebrex every day for most of my life."

He says he has had chronic pain, infection, fatigue and joint pain his whole adult life.

"All of my pain was relieved in four or five days," he says.

After two treatments, "Twenty years of pain were gone. No pain. It was the first time I slept through the night in years. My pain going away is a miracle."

Paul also talks about amazing mental clarity. "My brain lit up like a light bulb."

He talks about healing methods used by the Egyptians and about vitamin drips and liquid forms of minerals. This guy is so excited about being pain free he can probably talk me into anything.

He says, "I've worked with Dr. Mark Bartiss for a long time and trust him with my life."

I'm very excited to hear the treatments have worked for these two people.

I feel even better when Paul asks, "Do you think we can pray together?"

I'll admit I've been leaning on my faith a little more these days, so I say, "Sure."

His prayer is so good. He prays: "Lord, we glorify You and know You are all powerful. Lord, thank you for giving Dr. Bartiss the knowledge to help people. Lord, we know if we ask You the door will be opened. Lord, if it's your will, remove the cancer from Paula's body. Let every cancer cell be destroyed. Let Dr. Bartiss's hands be guided by You and be a source of healing. All this and more in Jesus' name. Amen."

The prayer is the icing on the cake.

It crosses my mind that Dr. Bartiss, of course, isn't going to have two people call me who have had bad experiences. Still, I'm excited to try something noninvasive that may help my immune system so that my body has a chance to heal itself.

My last appointment is with the surgeon. Dr. Daugherty is very respectful. He understands I want my immune system strong before I will even consider surgery.

He tells me, "I like doing surgery within four weeks of radiation to make it easier for me."

I appreciate his honesty.

He explains, "There is no scar tissue yet. Once scar tissue forms, it sometimes doesn't suture well and waiting too long might require a plastic surgeon to add new skin."

He gives me diagrams of the surgery.

I'm happy I'd taken a Xanax, or I'd be crying all over his desk. This is a life-changing operation.

While we're talking with the doctor, the receptionist comes into the doctor's office, harried, hurried and anxious that I quickly pick a date for surgery. Dr. Daugherty is in the middle of showing me how he'll rearrange all my organs and is explaining the new way I'm to relieve myself.

He tells the receptionist, "Give us a couple more minutes."

He shows me new and improved colostomy bags. He explains how advanced they'd become since he started his practice.

I'm in shock. I sit there just staring blankly as he goes on talking.

And there is that inner voice of mine, again speaking to me, saying, *I am not going to do this operation.*

Such an operation seems barbaric to me. All these years of technology and research and they can't figure out a better way of doing this?

I don't feel like I'm dying. I'm going to take my chances. I'm going to cash in my IRAs early, suffer the penalty and take my entire family on a nice vacation. If I'm going to leave this world this early, I'm going to have some fun first.

Just as I start to form a bucket list in my head, the receptionist comes into the office again.

With urgency, she says, "Dr. Daugherty has a vacation coming up. The doctor is accommodating you regarding which hospital you want to use. This is making scheduling very difficult. You have to make a decision about the surgery today."

She threw out the date of April 13. That's the date my mother died several years earlier.

I tell her, "That date is out of the question."

Whoa! Slow down. I can't take this pressure right now and this feels like a high-pressure sale.

I can't get it out of my head that Dr. Daugherty had said, "If you don't do surgery right away, it's been my experience that some people come back six months, one year, or even two years later to get the surgery."

To me that means I'm not in immediate danger of dying.

"Thank you for the information Dr. Daugherty. I will call to set the surgery appointment at a later date."

I pick up my portable seat cushion and Jack and I leave.

On the ride home, I remind Jack of a conversation we had had with Dr. Stevens when she told us, "One of my own family members who had breast cancer did not have an operation. Many years later, that same family member had rectal cancer and again would not have the operation. She lived into her 80's."

Dr. Stevens called that family member an anomaly.

Hey, that anomaly could be me too, right? Why not?

Five more days of chemotherapy and then I'm done.

Chapter 8   Looking For a Miracle

February 28, 2012: End of chemotherapy.

Woo-hoo!

As actor Matthew McConaughey said, "Alright, alright, alright!"

In the beginning, I had had a one-track mind and was committed to the chemo and radiation. Once I start something, I finish it.

Earlier, Lois gave me a copy of Suzanne Somers's book *Knockout*. It scared me so much that I couldn't continue reading it while undergoing conventional treatments. Clearly, the chemo and radiation are poison to my body.

I don't want that negative information floating around in my thoughts.

When I research anything about cancer treatments online, it's overwhelming and fills me with anxiety. There's so much information.

I had been told by medical and radiation oncologists that the one-two punch of chemo and radiation could possibly eliminate the cancer. I'd believed that and worked hard for it to become a reality. I've given conventional medicine all of January and February. I've put all of my positive energy into becoming cancer free by the end of February.

But, now, I'm open to all options.

I'm looking for the miracle.

I find it ironic that my last day of chemo is also my first alternative treatment with Dr. Bartiss.

It takes an hour to get to Bartiss' office. It's interesting how I'd always felt bad for Sarah and Rob because it took them an hour to travel to their radiation treatments. It's really not that bad. An hour gives me time to think, and I have a lot to think about.

Bartiss enters the treatment room wearing a Hawaiian shirt, jeans and orange sneakers. His casual attire helps relieve my white-coat syndrome. He's knowledgeable, likable and humorous. I find out that he's also an author, a lecturer and a medical writer. I want to be as comfortable as possible, because my rear was still hurting and I hate needles. I take a pain pill and a .25-milligram Xanax.

I feel only a pinch. It's a fascinating process. Dr. Bartiss blasts ozone into the saline solution and puts into the solution the blood he took from me. The blood passes through an ultraviolet machine and then back into my body through an intravenous tube. I'm making my own vaccine with my own blood.

I'm given ozone-infused olive oil to ease the radiation burns that are around my private areas. Within a couple days of applying the oil, the affected area is relieved. The itch stops and the burned skin begins to rejuvenate itself.

Leap day, February 29: A group of us goes to a wake and funeral Mass in Manhattan to pay last respects to our cousin's husband.

The Mass has my mind spinning again. The 100-year-old church is right across the street from the funeral parlor. It's nestled into the landscape of a Manhattan neighborhood. Once we pass through the large wooden Gothic doors, the first thing we see is an ornate baptismal font. The confessionals to the left have oversize carved wood doors with a small round light at the top that would turn red if the confessional is in use. There's a hollow feel in the gathering space and when we speak to each other we can detect a slight echo.

To deliver his homily from the carved marble pulpit, the priest has to climb several steps to reach the perch above the congregation.

This old church has my imagination exploding with negative cancer thoughts. *What will my funeral be like? Almost everyone here will be at my funeral. How will Katie handle my funeral? STOP IT! STOP IT!*

The burial is at Holy Cross Cemetery in Brooklyn, where many members of my mother's side of the family are buried. The weather is crazy, nasty, cold and rainy. All we need is wind, and that picks up while we're at the graveside.

After a short service, we go back to Manhattan to a Spanish restaurant that my cousin's husband liked.

Being in that old church reminds me of my Catholic school upbringing. Daily Mass was a requirement when we went to Sacred Heart School, which has one of the oldest churches in Trenton attached to it.

Old churches and funerals have a way of making you think about your own mortality, and Jack and I have had talks about quality-of-life issues and end-of-life issues.

When we have a moment alone, I tell Jack, "You know I'm willing to live with the decisions I make for myself."

He reassures me, "Nothing is going to happen to you. No matter what, I will always support you and stand by your decision, whatever it is. I love you. I'll always be here for you."

The one I worry about is Katie. She's not OK with what I'm doing, or should I say *not* doing. She thinks an operation is the answer. I feel Katie has been avoiding me.

When we do talk, she acts angry and says, "If you would just agree to have the operation, everything would be fine."

But that's not true. This is a major, life-changing operation, which may or may not help.

No one knows.

Not one doctor has given me a guarantee of anything. There are too many what-ifs.

All I know is that I feel too good to let myself be sliced up from under my breastbone to my pelvic area and then have my colon rearranged and my rectum taken out.

I'm not saying no to this operation; I'm just saying, "Let me try naturally."

If I need to do it, I will know I need to and God will guide me. I truly feel God will give me a sign.

I just hope that when I meet Him at the pearly gates, He doesn't say, "I sent you three surgeons and you said no to all of them."

I believe He will put the right people in my path at exactly the right time to help me heal myself.

Sometimes a challenge is put into your life to redirect you to a new path. I'm not sure why this is happening to me. I just hope God feels I have more work left to do here on Earth.

It's March 1 and Lois and Jack are with me for my second treatment. I feel great. I'm hopeful and happy that this treatment may cure the cancer. I want to avoid ever having to get cut up. NO CUTTING!

This time, Mark—Dr. Bartiss has asked me to call him Mark—adds some anti-inflammatory stuff to the intravenous tube.

He asks, "How are the burns on your butt doing?"

He wants to see my rear, so Lois comes with me to another room.

Mark tells Jack, "I'm going to see something you're never going to see."

I had previously told Mark, "Jack has never even seen me sitting on the toilet, never mind my burned-up butt."

When I tell them, "I can't see it well," they take a picture of my rear with my cell phone. Now we're all laughing.

Who does stuff like this?

Jack likes Mark because Mark says, "It's very important to keep intimacy a priority."

Apparently, illness can be hard on relationships.

I'm happy to hear Jack say, "Honey, don't worry, everything is OK in the intimacy department."

My sister says, "I told you Mark is different from the doctors you've been to lately."

"I kind of figured that out at our first meeting. On his desk sits a bomb with the letter *F* on top of it. F- bomb! And everyone around here is pretty comfortable using the *F* word."

Lois and I giggle the whole ride home. Lois wonders, "How much do you think a before-and-after picture of your ass would be worth to the medical community?"

Wow, what an unbelievable adventure I'm on. For this moment, right now, I'm happy to be able to laugh about the circumstances. I guess it helps that I read my affirmations every day and expect good things to happen to me.

One word can describe this past week: ITCHY! My butt itches, my hands itch and my feet itch. I'm told itching could be a minor side effect of the chemo pills. I have trouble sleeping because I can't find any cream that works to stop the itch. It's so not attractive scratching your ass.

I have a fiftieth birthday party to go to tonight: I've got to stop scratching.

An antihistamine finally gives me some relief.

My sisters continue to blow me away with their generosity.

They give up so much in order to help me.

They come up with funds when I need them.

They do research with a passion that takes a lot of time.

It all brings me to tears: happy tears.

God, too, is watching over me. Next week, Jack has a real estate closing whose fee will pay for my treatments for the next several months. The house in question has been sitting around on the market for a while. Now, all of a sudden, a buyer appears who wants to close in thirty days. And the commission is almost to the penny the amount needed for the treatments.

I don't think that's a coincidence. I prayed to God for help — specifically, to help me find the money to pay for these treatments and, *bam*, those prayers are being answered.

I do treatments three days a week right now. I'll try to get in as many treatments as possible before I do another PET scan. Besides a biopsy, a PET scan is the only way to find out whether the cancer is gone.

I have a lot of friends and family whose birthday parties are in March. This is good because as long as I'm busy, my fear stays under control.

St. Patrick's Day is also coming up, which always means a party. Everyone will come to our house for corned beef and cabbage. The food will be delicious, thanks to Jack.

Next up is the follow-up appointment with Dr. Rivers, the medical oncologist. The goal is to have her order a PET scan so I can find out whether the cancer is gone.

I'm feeling anxious.

Jack and I are sitting in the waiting area at Dr. Rivers's office. It's the first time I'm seeing her since completing the course of chemo and radiation. I know the cancer team is not happy that my name is not on the surgery schedule.

Dr. Rivers asks, "When is your surgery scheduled?"

"It's not scheduled."

"Why not?"

"I'm more afraid of the surgery than I am of the cancer. And don't you want to see whether the chemo and radiation have healed the cancer?"

"Not really. It doesn't matter to us. We feel you should have the surgery even if it's gone."

And she added something about so-called invisible cells that don't show up on any tests.

She's very understanding about my concerns about my immune system's not being up to par, yet I can tell she's not used to dealing with patients who don't do exactly what doctors tell them to do.

She starts to ask questions like, "What will it take for you to make a decision?"

Wow! Way to sell me that surgery, Doctor.

"Let's do a PET scan to see whether the cancer is still there," I say. "That will help me with my decision making."

Before ordering the test, she says: "I'm sure you've already been told, but I'm going to tell you again: If the cancer comes back, it will be very painful and the chemo more strenuous."

Wow! Way to scare the poop out of me.

A PET scan is ordered for April 18. Mission accomplished.

Dr. Rivers says, "Your cancer marker for the last PET scan was 12+. If it's a 2 this time, it could be inflammation."

I feel as if she's rooting for me at this point.

She also tells me about a fellow who didn't do the surgery. In fact, he did nothing — not even chemo or radiation. Three years later, he died of an illness completely unrelated to the cancer. They always say there's an exception to the rule. An anomaly.

Why can't *I* be that exception?

Chapter 9   Belief

Four months into this cancer diagnosis and I really feel good; I don't feel as if I have cancer. If they didn't show me the picture of the ugly tumor, I wouldn't believe it.

I'm happy and appreciating every day.

It's funny how once you think your time is limited, you appreciate everything more.

Jack and I are relaxing in the yard. It's dusk and the sun is setting, shining through the cracks of the stockade fence. It looks so beautiful. How many times had that very scene happened before?

Yet I appreciate it — and many other everyday things — more than I used to before the diagnosis.

Cancer has awakened me to many things I'd taken for granted.

I'm a lucky girl. Jack treats me like a princess. Every morning he prepares coffee, aloe vera, Echinacea tea, lemon water and veggies he juices fresh every day in the Vitamix blender. All of them delicious and healthy foods.

Time is moving quickly. Easter is right around the corner. Everyone will be at Lois' house. I look forward to seeing family.

He is risen. Thank you, Jesus, for all that you do for me. I love you more every day.

Our first time up to the mountains is great.

It's so peaceful before all the summer people come.

It's our place to recharge.

Before we leave, Jack assures me, "We'll have many more trips to our Eagle Lake getaway."

My stomach has been acting up and making a lot of noise. I put ozone-infused olive oil in me every night and I'm still doing ultraviolet ozone transfusions with Dr. Bartiss.

I'm anxious about having the PET scan on Wednesday.

I can't be near anything negative, but I guess I'm only human. I cried today because sometimes I'm scared.

Cancer thoughts get into my head, even though I do everything I can to dispel them. *I know God's in control and I trust Him. I just have to let go and believe He will take care of things.*

I pray a lot. I start the day with, "Angel of God, my Guardian dear, to whom God's love commits me here, ever this day be at my side, to light and guard, to rule and guide. Amen."

I'm in the middle of a Rosary novena to Our Lady. It requires praying the rosary every day for fifty-four days. The first twenty-seven days serve as a petition for asking for what I want. The second twenty-seven are in thanksgiving for what I already have.

Each day, I meditate on a different mystery.

Praying is very effective in keeping negative thoughts at bay and the beads passing through my fingers are very relaxing.

I pray to the Immaculate Heart of Mary. I pray to Our Lady of Lourdes. A friend of mine went to the grotto in Lourdes, France, where Saint Bernadette Soubirous, the young daughter of a poor miller, saw apparitions of the Blessed Virgin Mary. Young Bernadette was instrumental in the making of the Shrine of Our Lady of Lourdes, which five million people visit every year looking for a miracle.

My friend brought me back a beautiful glass bottle of holy water with an image of the grotto on it. When I notice the water is evaporating, I drink what is left of it.

To this day, that holy water bottle is on my nightstand.

I pray to Saint Peregrine, the patron saint of cancer patients, known for both his holiness and the miraculous healing he himself received. He was scheduled to have a leg amputated because of a cancerous growth, but the night before the surgery, he prayed for a healing and received a vision of Christ coming down from the cross to touch his leg, which completely healed it.

My favorite is still Saint Bernadette. Even though her story happened more than 150 years ago, Saint Bernadette had the same issues with conventional doctors and the Church as if they were happening today.

The conventional doctors wanted proof of the miracles, which they eventually got. The Church thought Bernadette was boastful and not too bright. Which was not true.

She was sickly and had a tough life.

Besides the remarkable story of the visions of the Immaculate Conception, another almost unbelievable story surrounding Saint Bernadette happened thirty years after her death: Her body was to be moved to another location and it was found to be in a perfectly preserved state. Her skin was hard but intact, and her color remanded. Today, Saint Bernadette's body can still be seen incorrupt in the chapel of Nevers in a glass casket, where she appears to be asleep.

Besides praying, I put positive affirmations in prominent spots so that I see them often throughout the day.

For instance, at the top of the pages of my journal I write, "This too shall pass" and "I expect good things to happen today."

And in my day planner I write, "I am a healthy and strong girl. No matter what, I'm going to be OK. I'm precious and infinitely loved more than I could possibly imagine. I bounce back quickly and I am resilient."

And here are other particular favorites: "Don't move the way fear makes you move. Move the way *love* makes you move. Move the way joy makes you move."

"The unconditional and perfect love of God neglects not one soul."

I'm not gonna let these negative thoughts get the best of me.

One more—I love this one too: "Everything the enemy has stolen, God is going to restore: the joy, the peace, the health, the dreams."

Somebody turned me on to Bruce Lipton, and I'm reading one of his books: *The Biology of Belief.* Listen to this—and I do believe it: "By speaking powerful positive words and thinking powerful positive thoughts, you absolutely can turn your body pH to a state of alkaline and reverse—yes, that's right, absolutely cure—virtually every disease in the body, all with the power of your mind."

I have a busy day. PET scan at 8:30 a.m., lunch with Debbie at 1, massage at 4:30 and a 7:30 church seminar.

Staying busy is good.

I make it through the PET scan.

Lunch with Debbie is great: risotto, vichyssoise and a nice Malbec. Home in time for a nap before my massage.

When I wake up, my stomach has cramps; I felt them during the massage. They get worse as the night goes on, but I still go to the talk at the church.

I have to do the citrus citrate and a Dulcolax for my visit to Dr. Bartiss tomorrow. The cramps started early; maybe it's only gas or maybe I ate something bad at lunch. I didn't sleep well. The citrate cleaned me out, but the cramps didn't go away.

Maybe it's just PET scan nerves.

I'm shocked that Dr. Bartiss's office already has the PET scan results. I'm also crushed that the cancer marker has gone only from 11.9 to 11.3. Another marker has lowered from 26 to 18.8.

I really don't understand what it actually means.

Mark sees I'm visibly upset, so he spins it as positively as he can, "The fact of the matter is, it's lower and it's moving in the right direction."

He even points out, "The second marker is 30 percent lower than last time, which is a good deal lower."

"But I expected it to be completely GONE. No more cancer."

We talk about a game plan for tracking progress. There is no more blood. Mark does another digital, looking for a tumor, and he can't find one. Every one of the other doctors led me to believe the tumor can see light. He went in 7 centimeters, and no tumor.

Mark makes me feel he is vested in helping me become cancer free.

"I'm going to a convention in a couple of weeks," he says. "I want to ask the experts in natural cures for cancer, face-to-face, what we should be doing next."

"Can I have your permission to present your case at the convention."

"Absolutely."

I do treatments once a month, now. Next week, I have a consultation with Kristen, the house dietitian for Dr. Bartiss's office.

The cancer is still there, but I'm upping my game.

I will do whatever it takes to get rid of this cancer.

I still believe my body can and will heal itself naturally.

Chapter 10   Suzette

Negative cancer thoughts are getting the best of me. My friend Patti suggests I see Suzette, a creative visualization facilitator.

"Suzette is helping people lose weight by hypnotizing them. Maybe she could help you with your 'stinkin thinkin'," Patti says.

Because my cancer budget is depleted, I tell her, "I can't come up with funds right now."

"Not to worry: the beauty of this is that she can't charge. She's still in training, so she would only be practicing her skills on you."

As my sister, Susan, would say, "That's not odd; that's God."

We meet at a studio that has been set up in a detached garage at Suzette's house. Everything needed for relaxation is there. I make myself comfortable in a cozy recliner. Suzette offers me a plush comforter to keep me warm. Soft music is playing in the background.

Suzette asks, "OK, what are you trying to accomplish here? How can I help you?"

"I was diagnosed with cancer in late December. Until recently, I've been very positive. But now I'm completely overwhelmed with fear. I hope you can help me get back on track. I did chemo and radiation, but I put the brakes on the conventional doctors when they told me my only option for survival was a permanent colostomy operation. I don't believe that will cure me. I believe my body is capable of healing itself. I'm working with an alternative doctor and I'd like to try to heal naturally."

"Wow, that's an amazing story. I love that you're trying to heal naturally. I, too, believe the body can heal itself. You can do this. I'm in it for the duration. I'll help you."

Suzette has this big amazing smile that is accented with ruby red lipstick. Her beautiful eyes look over the top of black-and-white-polka-dot eyeglasses. She has short, cropped hair and appears to be my age – give or take a couple years. She looks right at me while I'm talking. I can tell Suzette is interested in everything I have to say. She's fun, quirky and authentic.

"Normally, I'm very positive, but lately, negative cancer thoughts been getting the best of me and I can't seem to shake them," I offer.

"We're going to work on your thoughts. Now let's get started."

Suzette's voice alone can make you feel relaxed. "Now, in a few minutes I will count from ten down to one. As I count, I want you to imagine— I want you to think like you're at the top. With each step leading down—ten—imagine taking that first step down, relaxing more and more as you do. Just feeling and being completely calm—nine, eight, seven. Calmer and calmer—four— drifting deeper and deeper—three, two—one. You're completely relaxed."

Deep in the relaxed state of creative visualization, when asked to think back to my earliest memories, tears start to leak from my eyes. Even though I have happy childhood memories, I find out that I hold on to negative feelings about being the only kid in my class who comes from, as they used to call it, a "broken" home.

"As a kid, I remember the teacher called me aside to make sure I was OK, because I came from a 'broken' home."

"I remember laughing it off and thinking, my family isn't broken. I see lots of families that seem way more broken than mine."

Although my parents divorced when I was around six, I had a great childhood. I was the middle sister of three girls. I have memories of stuff happening around the time of the divorce, but I always felt loved. My mother remarried and our new father accepted us as his own. In my mid-teens, my brother was born. We never used terms like *stepfather* or *half-brother*; we were just a regular family.

Being hypnotized is like being in a dream like state—not awake yet not fully asleep—and the brain slows down to a theta state. When the mind is in such a trance-like state, the conscious mind is not paying full attention and the subconscious mind is more receptive to suggestion.

My first hypnosis session goes well – until the ride home.

Along a country road, I hear a noise that sounds like I ran over something huge. Then the car just stops running. As luck would have it, two good ole' boys, both of whom knew about cars, are in the pickup truck behind me. They stop to help.

"Sounds to me like the transmission," one of them said, as I'm fishing in my pocketbook for my AAA card.

It starts to drizzle as I wonder aloud, "That sounds expensive."

"I live two minutes up the road: the farm on the right," the man says. "I can be back in no time with my flatbed and get you to the shop much faster than if you waited for AAA."

"Sure, thanks," I say as I text Jack on my cell phone to let him know about my situation.

At least I'm relaxed, because life sure can get crazy.

My second session with Suzette reveals that I use laughter as a defense mechanism. As in all families, my family has had its disagreements and arguments with one another, but nothing any other family hasn't experienced, too. If Irish tempers flared, I was the kid in the family who would think it was hysterically funny and laugh it off.

I married in my late 20s and had a beautiful baby girl. Within five years of Katie's birth, her father and I grew apart. Since I had been a child of divorce, I thought I, myself, would never divorce.

Well, never say never. Divorce has been probably one of the hardest things I've had to go through in my life – second only to my mother's death and this cancer.

I find out I'm holding on to guilt about leaving my first husband. Although I did what was right for me at the time, I wish he hadn't had to get hurt along the way. But I don't regret doing it.

I have to let go of the guilt.

I learn that I have resentments I have to let go of and to forgive all the people who hurt me.

I was good at the forgiveness part, but I'm still holding on to the hurts.

I have to consciously learn to let go of the hurts.

Funny thing is, I didn't even know I was holding on to all this stuff. It wasn't until I entered a deeply relaxed state that all of those thoughts surfaced. I don't know how or where the thoughts come from.

But they come.

I have to forgive not only others; I have to forgive myself.

To help me reach a peaceful state, Suzette uses visualization, stories, metaphors and relaxation techniques. Once I'm in a state of trance, she makes suggestions to help me accomplish the goals: letting go of guilt, letting go of fear, letting go of resentments.

When I drop my car off for repair of the transmission, the shop owner says, "This is a big job. You also need two new front tires. And when we're done with *your car,* you have to bring in Jack's car for shocks." *Cha-ching.*

So, we are officially a one car family this week.

Today Jack drops me off at Suzette's and we'll pick up his car after my session. I look forward to having my independence back. It's not easy sharing a car when we're each running in opposite directions.

Suzette introduces me to a Louise Hay recording called "Cancer: Discovering Your Healing Power." I listen to this recording at least once a day, sometimes twice a day. It's filled with forgiveness techniques.

One of the lessons is to look in the mirror and tell yourself, "I love you; I really, really love you."

No problem—I think I have great self-esteem. I do love myself.

Well, try it yourself.

The first time I look directly into my own eyes in the mirror and say, "I love you; I really, really love you," it feels weird. I'm uncomfortable saying that to myself, but I continue until it becomes easy to say.

I'm also learning I have to love myself exactly as I am.

Suzette and I become fast friends. Suzette is very good at what she does. The work she's doing with me is priceless.

I don't think she'll ever truly realize how much she's helping me.

I'm learning how to handle life's stresses.

Suzette tells me, "When stress happens, you can choose how you're going to react."

Hypnosis is effective in changing negative habits and limiting beliefs. It's a peaceful way to create change.

One of the benefits of hypnosis is relief of stress because it's so relaxing.

We go to pick up Jack's car and are shocked to see that the front end is crashed in. Apparently, someone had taken the car for a joyride and brought it back smashed up. I figure only a foolish kid would do something like that. We had given the keys to one of the workers who was the only one there all night.

When the cops come, the worker says, "The car never left the station while I was here."

C'mon. Do you think we're stupid? And why is it that criminals have all the rights? Even though everything pointed to this kid, even though he was the only one with access to the key, even though all the circumstantial evidence pointed directly at him, the windup is that because no one saw him in the car, the police aren't permitted to fingerprint him to prove he's the culprit. We needed witnesses.

Then my sister Susan sides with the kid. She says, "Paula, you're lucky because you have Jack and a second car. Life is easy for you."

"Yeah, right, my car just got stolen, someone crashed it and I'm dealing with cancer. I don't need this added stress."

Susan adds, "The kid will have to live with his guilt."

I was not feeling sorry for this kid.

The next day, while Jack is speaking to the owner of the shop, the kid approaches Jack and apologizes. He confesses to taking the car and crashing it.

"I'm sorry, mister. When I saw the cops, I just got scared."

Susan is right about his feeling guilty.

The young man told Jack, "I'll pay $100 a week till the deductible is covered."

That's right: I'm calling him a young man now.

Good grief. You can't make this stuff up, but thanks to Suzette, I'm learning how to relax and let things go. It's an ongoing process. I have to consciously practice relaxation daily. There's always going to be something to stress about.

Suzette is teaching me self-hypnosis. Her upbeat energy and her belief that the body can heal itself are the kinds of characteristics I want surrounding me. Self-hypnosis is a great segue into meditation and both help with relaxation.

I consider Suzette one of the people God put in my path to help me heal.

I'm also grateful to the two-good-ole' boys who rescued me on that country road the day my car broke down.

Even the fellow who owned up to his wrongdoing in crashing Jack's car has a lesson for me to learn.

Maybe Susan is right.

I do have it made. I am lucky, or maybe I have guardian angels watching over me.

Chapter 11 You Can't Scare Me!

I'm on the phone with Kristen the dietitian from Dr. Bartiss's office for an hour and a half today.

"It sounds like Jack is doing a fantastic job with all the home-cooked meals. It's great you have a supportive husband," she offers.

"Oh, I know how lucky I am. I could never do all of this alone. I feel that Jack's support in the kitchen is keeping me alive."

Kristen advises: "I want you to stay away from all processed foods. You must detox your body with a three-day organic juice cleanse."

She also suggests red clover herbs made into tea.

"You can get store-bought red clover tea, but picking it in the wild is better for you, although you have to make sure you pick it where there are no pesticides."

It sounds like the Essiac tea Susan gives me. We talk about spirulina, which is seaweed and algae. It's similar to the E3Live that Susan gives me. Susan is very helpful with her cancer research.

Bottom line, by the end of the conversation, Kristen says, "I want you to try a totally organic vegetarian diet for at least one month, starting with the three-day juice-only organic cleanse. Recipes are on the way via e-mail."

I like Kristen. She sounds young but also as if she knows her stuff.

Dr. Bartiss tells me, "Kristen has worked successfully with other patients who have colon cancer, so pay attention to what she says."

I can have eggs — organic and preferably free-range because she says she'd like the eggs to come from happy chickens playing in the sunshine, receiving their vitamin D naturally from the sun and eating happy seeds and grass with no pesticides.

Jack's life-long interest in healthy lifestyles will make the transition to healthier eating habits easier for us than starting from scratch.

Jack's love of cooking started early. On my kitchen windowsill, I keep a picture of him around two years old sitting on an aluminum kitchen table stirring a bowl of homemade cookie dough.

Coming from an Italian family, he watched his *nonna* and *his* mother make homemade meals daily. Three generations lived in the house Jack's grandfather built in 1907 on Whittaker Avenue in Chambersburg for the family.

Jack loves to tell stories: "My mom would give me fifty cents or a dollar and I'd walk to Tammaro's grocery store to get a bag filled with mixed vegetables for making soup or stew.

Back then, everything was fresh, local and pesticide free. We were eating organic and didn't even know it."

After college, Jack joined the U.S. Army. That's where his enthusiasm for cooking really grew.

Army food.

While everyone else was eating in the mess hall, Jack made friends with the cook and could prepare food for himself.

Always interested in health and fitness, Jack was a runner. He even ran marathons. In the late '70s early '80s, he wrote for the local newspaper, the Trentonian, a runner's column called 'Beyond Jogging'.

Also in the '70s, Jack opened a vitamin store in Trenton. It was a risky venture because the FDA and the pharmaceutical companies were trying to get control of vitamin sales. They wanted vitamins to require prescriptions so that people would have to see a doctor to get them.

But because most vitamins are plant-based, they're considered a food.

And the pharmaceutical companies have not yet reached their goal.

Dr. Bartiss will be home from his convention tomorrow. He's talking to natural-healing doctors from all over the world. I feel I'm leading a double life: one with alternative medicine and one with conventional medicine.

In a couple of days, I'll see Dr. Stevens again. My game plan for that meeting is to ask her to please have patience, to have a little faith and to be positive about the decisions I make for myself because I'm the only one who will have to live with the consequences. And for me, a permanent colostomy bag would be one huge consequence.

I want to talk about the PET scan results because I don't know what all the numbers mean. I also want to talk about the best way to check my progress.

A quarterly colonoscopy maybe?

Jack and I are at the 10 o'clock appointment with the radiation oncologist. Dr. Stevens is disappointed that I'm not doing the operation recommended by the cancer team, which consists of Dr. Rivers, the medical oncologist, Dr. Daugherty, the colorectal surgeon, and Dr. Stevens.

When I ask for an explanation of the results of the PET scan, Dr. Stevens says, "I don't want to comment because it's not my area of expertise."

"Who then?"

"Whoever ordered it."

She knew that Dr. Rivers the medical oncologist had ordered the test. I asked about the PET scan only because even though it had been performed a month ago, I never received a phone call with the results.

Yet Dr. Bartiss's office spoke to me about the results the very next day after the procedure.

I figure Dr. Stevens can help me with the PET scan because she's part of the cancer team.

But I find out that neither Dr. Stevens nor Dr. Rivers received a copy of the results.

Then Dr. Stevens becomes combative, saying, "Normally, a PET scan wouldn't be ordered so soon. Dr. Rivers ordered it at your request."

But wait a minute: I'm the patient. If that test shouldn't have been ordered, wouldn't it be the doctor's decision and not mine?

Jack makes sure we get copies of all test results.

"Here's a copy of the recent PET scan for your file."

It doesn't seem to matter to Dr. Stevens that she now has a copy of the PET scan.

Then it hits me: I realize that the results of the test don't matter to them. Their only goal is to get me into the operating room.

Dr. Stevens says: "Any other doctor would be done with you once you choose not to do the surgery. No doctor would stick with you. Any doctor would just walk out. As your friend and as your doctor, you have to listen to me. If you were my family member, I would be much more persistent about your getting the surgery because you're playing with your life. Because you're choosing not to get the surgery, you need a doctor who will follow your cancer with a scope periodically. And you'll need to get a referral from your primary."

All of a sudden, the doctor I think I have such a great relationship with turns on me. For the past five months, I've dealt with these three doctors, now she wants me to go back to my primary, start over and find yet another doctor?

She also suggests I see a gastroenterologist.

I may be mistaken, but I think I've just been shown the door.

I speak to the office manager at Dr. Bartiss' office. "Hi, Lena, I want to learn what Mark found out at the convention."

"Mark has to let all the information sink in. Your file is on his desk. He'll call you soon."

Jack and I go to a chamber of commerce business luncheon and the first person we bump into is a friend who is an administrator at the hospital where my cancer team is affiliated. We have a long-story-short conversation about what's been happening. He makes a few phone calls and now we're meeting with Dr. Kerry Logan, a colorectal specialist.

Everything's easier when you know somebody.

Dr. Logan is to do an evaluation. This may be the best way to follow my progress and to see whether the tumor continues to shrink.

I give Dr. Logan the short version of the past six months, adding how I feel about the surgery.

I tell her, "I would like to try clean eating for six months to see whether that will keep the cancer from spreading and possibly shrink the tumor."

"I don't believe that school of thought, but let's do a colonoscopy to see what's happening," she says.

Her words and manner are kind and gentle, but I can tell she, too, thinks surgery is my best option.

She asks: "Do you have kids? Do you want to be at their weddings? Do you want to know your grandchildren?"

I think to myself, *I don't see what that line of questioning has to do with following my progress. And I don't appreciate it.*

"My mother was only fifty-one years old when she passed away," Dr. Logan says. "Her death is one of the reasons I decided to pursue a career in medicine."

It's a sad story, but I'm sticking to my guns and following the diet the dietitian has prescribed. I think I can keep my colon healthy naturally.

Dr. Logan orders a colonoscopy, and I've already planned a follow-up visit to go over the results.

Meanwhile, Jack and I go to a business expo. Jack meets Dr. Steuber, an acupuncturist. At Dr. Steuber's booth, he does a pulse test on the inside of the forearm. He moves his thumb and pointer finger up and down the inside of Jack's forearm, checking targeted pulse points. Then he talks to him about his health, saying, "You may have cholesterol and arthritis issues."

This is true.

Jack is so impressed with the procedure that he encourages me to see what Dr. Steuber might say about my health, but I'm skeptical. It seems like he's a health fortune-teller.

I make sure I don't say anything that could give him a clue that I have any health issues.

Then to my amazement, he tells me, "You have issues in your pelvic area." He doesn't mention anything specific, but he does say, "Something is definitely happening in that area."

He talks about the two-thousand years' acupuncture has been in use and its benefits, and gives me an informational brochure and a gift certificate for a free evaluation.

Jack and I think it's very interesting that this doctor hit the nail on the head regarding each of us.

By the way, Dr. Steuber's office is in the same building complex as Dr. Logan's. It's a small world.

I make it through another colonoscopy. I'm in this hospital way too often. I recognize and know the names of some of the nurses.

Even through the grogginess of anesthesia, I can see the tumor has shrunk considerably. The doctor doesn't seem as excited as Jack and me about how small the tumor looks. It doesn't matter to us what she thinks.

We can't wipe the smiles off our faces!

At the follow-up appointment, Dr. Logan keeps us for two long hours trying to convince me surgery is my only choice. We re-discuss what we talked about at our previous meeting.

"I'm thrilled with the tumor shrinkage," I say: "I'm very excited about sticking to my new diet so we can see whether it results in more shrinkage in the following six months."

Dr. Logan's stance is, "Diet will do nothing to improve your cancer diagnosis."

"It'll be great for you to see the difference six months from now," I say.

She counters: "I'm not interested in learning whether diet makes a difference. There have been no clinical trials proving diet will affect your cancer diagnosis."

When Dr. Logan sees I'm not changing my mind about the surgery, she raises the bar by looking right at Jack and saying: "If something happens to Paula, you'd better be willing to accept your daughter's resentment. What if Katie never forgives you for not pushing harder and not putting more pressure on Paula to have the operation?"

Are you kidding me? This is terrible. It blows my mind that she threw Katie into the mix.

Since when did they start teaching emotional blackmail at med school.

I'm also told: "The tumor is going to grow. You must undergo surgery while you're young and healthy. You're at the best you're going to be, and then, all of a sudden, the bottom will fall out. You're putting yourself at risk and you'd better be ready to die!"

I sit there numb. I keep my cool, though, because I want to check my progress with another colonoscopy in six months.

Having Jack with me keeps me strong.

I still have that visual in my head of how much smaller the tumor is, but I don't want to burn bridges. At the same time, scare tactics do not work on me. In fact, they do the complete opposite: *they make me determined to heal naturally!*

In the past six months, no one has given me any guarantees. Now, for sure, according to them, the tumor is going to grow.

I don't believe that.

My new diet is helping my body get into balance so that it can heal itself.

I leave there and go straight to the acupuncturist to make my first six appointments.

I want to align myself with positive professionals who believe I can help myself naturally.

Chapter 12   Jack's Chapter and Recipes

Today I'm making homemade escarole and bean soup for lunch, and for dinner gluten-free bucatini pasta with my mom's meat sauce recipe, meatballs and a salad.

For me, cooking is relaxation. I enjoy being in the kitchen, whether it's to make a James Beard recipe or something I create myself; I'm at home in a kitchen. Sometimes I'm alone or Paula is here to help me.

I'm a self-taught cook. I never attended a cooking class — just trial and error. Watching my Nonna and my mother cook all those years has stuck with me.

Paula and I have always eaten well, I thought. We eat very few processed foods, rarely fast foods and, for me, never any soft drinks. I prefer beer or water. We always like things fresh. My grandfather Prospero had a garden at our home in Trenton and it always included a fig tree or two. My dad continued the tradition and I still have a small garden.

When we discover Paula's cancer, we decide to go all organic, with non-genetically-modified-organism (GMO) foods. My garden is organic, but I can't produce enough food for us.

We discover Sandbrook Meadow Farm in Stockton, New Jersey. It's a community-supported-agriculture farm that is GMO free and organic. From June through December, we get plenty of fresh organic produce, herbs and weeds from Sandbrook. For instance, purslane is a weed that grows wild all over the place. It is delicious and its succulent leaves have more omega-3 fatty acids than some of the fish oils do. It grows abundantly at the farm and we can pick all we want for free.

Another weed we've grown to enjoy is red clover, which has a delicate flavor. We brew and enjoy it hot and cold as a tea. Because of its popularity with bees, it's naturally sweet, so you don't even have to use honey. Red clover has a celebrated reputation for its health benefits as a blood purifier, specifically for the potential treatment of colon cancer.

Kristen, Dr. Bartiss' dietitian, told us that the best way to get red clover is the wild plant. So, one sunny, beautiful day in June, when the wild clover is in full bloom, we find a field of it. Paula and I spend several hours in the clean fresh air picking red clover blooms. We fill a pillowcase with them. We dry the harvest naturally and then pack it away in mason jars. When we begin making tea, we can hardly believe the delicious taste. No sweetener is needed. The bees have done their job. In Shakespearean times, red clover was known as honey stalks. Now every spring we look for wild clover in untreated fields and pick to our hearts' content.

A daily staple in our diet is juice, not from a plastic bottle or from concentrate, but juice freshly made from fruits and vegetables. We use a Vitamix to make our juices and our basic recipe is simple:

2 cups of coconut water
1 rib of celery
¼ cucumber
1 piece of ginger (about ¾ to 1 inch)
½ lemon (remove pits)
1 apple (remove seeds)
2 or 3 kale or collard or Swiss chard leaves (stem removed)

After that you can get creative. The list is endless. Add fresh or frozen blueberries, strawberries, mangoes, carrots, beets, avocados, pineapples, asparagus, kiwi; just experiment to find out what your taste buds prefer. Better yet, pick up a book on juicing to get great advice.

One thing to remember: Always buy organic. In all of the recipes that follow, we strongly suggest the ingredients be organic. Sometimes organic might not be available, so you may have to use conventional or substitute something else, but do get creative.

Why is organic so important? Simple. It's good for people and good for the environment. Organic farmers work with nature to build rich, healthy soil and preserve biodiversity and critical water resources. Organic farming also means crops are grown without the use of genetic engineering (GMO's) or synthetic pesticides and fertilizers. By eating organic, we not only are limiting our exposure to those synthetic chemicals, but we're also respecting and utilizing nature's rich ecosystem. Organic food is the way food should be.

Here's a list to help you with your shopping. The Dirty Dozen should *always* be organic. With the Clean Fifteen, you can buy conventional. For everything not mentioned, use your discretion.

THE DIRTY DOZEN (+)
1. Apples
2. Peaches
3. Nectarines
4. Strawberries
5. Grapes
6. Celery
7. Spinach
8. Sweet bell peppers
9. Cucumbers
10. Cherry tomatoes
11. Snap peas
12. Potatoes
13. Hot peppers
14. Kale/collard greens

THE CLEAN FIFTEEN
1. Avocados
2. Sweet corn(non-GMO)
3. Pineapples
4. Cabbage
5. Sweet peas (frozen)
6. Onions
7. Asparagus
8. Mangoes
9. Papayas (non-GMO)
10. Kiwi
11. Eggplant
12. Grapefruit
13. Cantaloupe
14. Cauliflower
15. Sweet potatoes

So here are some of our favorite recipes.
For measurements: T = tablespoon, t = teaspoon, C = cup

BASIC VINAGRETTE
3 T organic olive oil
3 T organic raw unfiltered apple cider vinegar
1 T Dijon mustard
¼ t sea salt
¼ t organic black pepper
¼ t minced organic garlic from the USA, not China

Combine all ingredients in a glass jar, shake to combine and serve on salads.

Variations: Add crumbled blue cheese or your fa ⌐
herbs or spices.

RANCH AVOCADO DRESSING
  1 large avocado
  2 t fresh lemon juice
  ½ C plain yogurt*
  1 t hot sauce
  ¼ C organic olive oil
  2 cloves organic garlic, minced and from the USA, not
  China
  ½ t sea salt

Combine all ingredients in a glass jar, shake to combine
and serve on salad.

*We use plain organic raw milk yogurt, available in Pennsylvania but
not in New Jersey; certain organizations are working to make raw milk
available in New Jersey.

PEAR, BLUE CHEESE AND WALNUT SALAD
  ½ C organic olive oil
  Juice of ½ lemon
  ¼ t honey (local is best)
  ¼ t sea salt
  ¼ t organic pepper
  2 C organic baby spinach
  1 Bosc pear, quartered and thinly sliced
  ¼ C crumbled blue cheese
  ¼ C toasted walnuts

Whisk together oil, lemon juice, honey, salt and pepper.
Toss spinach and pear with dressing and sprinkle with
blue cheese and walnuts.

BLACK BEAN, CORN, AND TOMATO SALAD WITH CHILI LIME VINAIGRETTE

2 C organic black beans, rinsed and drained

1 C organic corn kernels (non-GMO)

1 C coarsely chopped organic greens (Use any combination of lettuce, kale, watercress, spinach, purslane, or spring mix.)

1 large ripe tomato, diced

3 organic green onions, thinly sliced

Chili Lime Vinaigrette

¼ C organic olive oil

2 T freshly squeezed lime juice

1 T Dijon mustard

1 t pure organic ground chili powder

½ t ground organic cumin

¼ t ground organic turmeric

¼ t sea salt

Combine in a large bowl the beans, corn, greens, tomato and green onions. In a small bowl, whisk together all vinaigrette ingredients. Pour over salad, toss to coat and serve chilled or at room temperature.

ROASTED TOMATO SALAD

Sandbrook Meadow Farm grows about seven or eight varieties of heirloom grape and cherry tomatoes, which makes this a show stopping addition to any meal.

8 C heirloom grape and cherry tomatoes

6 cloves organic garlic, cut in thin slices and from the USA, not China

1 T organic olive oil

2 T organic balsamic vinegar

½ t sea salt

¼ t organic black pepper
2–4 ounces of fresh mozzarella, cut into ½-inch cubes
10–12 fresh basil leaves, thinly sliced

Preheat oven to 350 degrees. Mix in a large bowl the tomatoes, garlic, oil, vinegar, salt and pepper. Using aluminum foil, make 4 pouches and divide the tomato mixture among the pouches. Fold pouches closed and pierce each pouch with a knife several times. Place pouches on a baking tray and roast for 20 minutes. Remove from oven, carefully open pouches and drain excess liquid. Place ½–1 ounce of cheese in each pouch, close pouch and continue to roast for 5 minutes. Let cool 3–5 minutes. Serve with sliced basil leaves.

GREEN BEAN AND TOMATO SALAD

Again, freshly picked green beans from the farm make a flavorful use of peak summer produce.

1 pound green beans, trimmed and cut into 2-inch pieces
2 pounds tomatoes, seeded and cut into ½-inch thick pieces
5 T organic balsamic vinegar
2 t organic garlic, minced and from the USA, not China
½ t sea salt
½ t organic black pepper
1 anchovy fillet, minced
3 T organic olive oil

Add green beans to a large pot of boiling water and cook 3–5 minutes until tender crisp. Drain and rinse in cold water to stop further cooking. Add tomatoes to green beans. Combine remaining ingredients in a glass jar and shake to combine. Pour over green bean and tomato mixture to coat.

ESCAROLE AND BEAN SOUP

So good and so easy.

   2 t organic olive oil
   1 C organic onions, chopped
   1 T organic garlic, minced and from the USA, not China
   4 C organic vegetable broth
   2 15-ounce cans organic cannellini beans, rinsed and
   drained
   4 C organic escarole, chopped
   Organic black pepper
   Grated Parmesan

Heat oil in large saucepan over medium-high heat. Add onions and garlic. Cook 5–7 minutes until tender, but do not brown. Add broth and beans; bring to a boil for 5 minutes. Stir in escarole and cook until escarole wilts, 4–6 minutes. Sprinkle with pepper and Parmesan.

WINTER VEGETABLE SOUP

This vegetable soup uses whole foods and spices that offer surprising health benefits for the entire family. Work together in the kitchen, chopping, stirring and improvising with whatever you have in your pantry and fridge.

   1 large organic onion
   2 large organic carrots
   3 organic celery ribs
   2 T organic olive oil
   2 cloves organic garlic, chopped and from the USA, not
   China
   2 t ground organic turmeric
   ½ t organic black pepper
   ½ t organic ground cayenne
   1 t organic dried oregano
   1 t organic dried basil
   ½ t organic dried thyme

2–4 t sea salt

4 quarts organic chicken broth

1 inch piece of organic ginger, finely grated

2 boneless, skinless, chicken breasts (free-range and antibiotic and hormone free)

½ pound mushrooms (shiitake, oyster, baby bella as available)

1 cloves organic garlic, grated and from the USA, not China

1 bunch flat-leaf Italian parsley, chopped

1 pound organic kale, Swiss chard, or baby spinach (as available)

Dice the onion, carrots and celery. Heat oil in large soup pot. Add the diced vegetables and gently sauté without browning, about 5–7 minutes. When onions become translucent, add the garlic and herbs and spices. Stir the mixture, heating it for 2–3 minutes. Add broth and grated ginger. Cube the chicken breast meat and add to the pot. Slice the mushrooms and add to the pot. Let soup simmer for 15 minutes and add the last grated clove of garlic to the soup. Add the parsley and any other chopped greens you like. Let the soup continue cooking until the greens have wilted. Serve and enjoy the healthy benefits of this wonderful soup.

CARAMELIZED ONION AND ASPARAGUS FRITTATA

1 t organic olive oil

2 large onions, finely chopped

12 fresh asparagus spears, trimmed

4 large eggs (from free-range chickens)

3 large egg whites (from free-range chickens)

¼ t sea salt

¼ t organic black pepper

¼ t organic turmeric powder
Coarsely chopped fresh organic parsley

Heat oil in ovenproof skillet (we like old cast iron skillets). Add onion and cook over moderate heat, stirring, about 2 minutes. Reduce heat to low and cook, stirring frequently, until onion is browned, about 25–30 minutes. Cook asparagus in boiling water about 3–5 minutes, until tender, and drain and set aside. Preheat broiler. In a bowl, whisk eggs, egg whites and 1 T of water. Season with salt, pepper and turmeric powder. Pour egg mixture over hot onions in skillet and let set for 1 minute. Cover and cook until eggs are set around the edges, 2–4 minutes. Arrange asparagus on top of the frittata, place skillet under the broiler and cook 30–60 seconds, or until omelet puffs up and is slightly browned. Sprinkle with chopped parsley and serve.

JACK'S AWARD-WINNING SWEETHEART CHILI*
2 t organic olive oil
½ pound organic yellow onions
1 pound hot Italian sausage, removed from casing
2-3 pounds ground beef (free-range and antibiotic-free)
2 T organic black pepper
1 6-ounce can organic tomato paste
3 T organic garlic, minced and from the USA, not China
1 t ground cumin
3 t plain chili powder
2 T Dijon mustard
1 t sea salt
1 T dried organic basil
1 T dried organic oregano
1 35-ounce can of diced imported Italian-style plum tomatoes (non-GMO)
½ C dry red wine
1 T fresh lemon juice

2 T fresh dill, chopped
2 T fresh Italian flat-leaf parsley, chopped
4 cans (1 each) organic dark red kidney beans, pinto beans, garbanzo beans, and black beans, drained and rinsed
1 T Valentina Salsa Picante (also serve at the table)
2 cans pitted black olives, drained

Heat oil in large soup pot. Add onion and cook over low heat until tender but not browned, about 10 minutes. Crumble sausage and beef into pot and cook over medium-high heat until all meats are well browned, stirring frequently. Lower heat and stir in pepper, tomato paste, garlic, cumin, chili powder, mustard, salt, basil and oregano. Add tomatoes, wine, lemon juice, dill, parsley, drained beans and Valentina Salsa Picante. Stir well to combine. Simmer 30 minutes to blend flavors. Taste to adjust seasonings. Add olives and simmer for an additional 15 minutes to heat. Serve in bowls, either as is or over whole-grain rice. Serve with bowls of sour cream, chopped onions, grated cheese and Valentina Salsa Picante for those who want to add more heat.

*Jack's Sweetheart Chili won first place in a chili cook-off at the HOB (Heart of Bordentown) Tavern in Bordentown, New Jersey.

PAULA'S FAVORITE GOULASH
2 pounds ground beef (free-range and antibiotic free)
2 medium organic onions, chopped
3 cloves organic garlic, minced and from the USA, not China
2 C filtered water or organic vegetable or beef broth
2 15-ounce cans organic tomato sauce
2 15-ounce cans organic diced tomatoes
½ t sea salt

¼ t organic black pepper
3 bay leaves
3 T tamari (gluten-free soy sauce, non-GMO)
2 C whole-grain elbow macaroni

In a large pot, cook beef over medium heat until browned. Add onion and garlic and sauté until transparent. Add the water or broth, tomato sauce, diced tomatoes, salt, pepper, bay leaves and tamari. Simmer for 15–20 minutes. Add macaroni and simmer for an additional 20 minutes or until macaroni is tender. Remove bay leaves before serving.

VEGETARIAN RISOTTO WITH FRESH ASPARAGUS
3 C organic vegetable broth
2 t organic olive oil
1/3 C diced organic onions
1 C Arborio rice
1 C asparagus, cut into 2-inch pieces
½ C freshly grated Parmesan
¼ t sea salt
¼ t organic black pepper
1 C asparagus, cut into 2-inch pieces

Heat the broth and keep hot over low heat. In a separate pot, heat olive oil over medium heat. Add onion and cook until translucent, 5 minutes. Add rice to onion mixture, turn heat to low and stir. Add about 1 C hot broth to rice mixture and stir until absorbed. Continue adding broth 1 C at a time, stirring; let rice absorb broth before adding more broth. While risotto is cooking, blanch asparagus in boiling water until tender, about 2–3 minutes, and drain. Reserve cooking liquid for soup base. The risotto is cooked when it's creamy on the outside and slightly firm in the center, about 20–25 minutes. Stir in half the Parmesan and half the asparagus. Season with salt and pepper. Serve in a large bowl and sprinkle with remaining asparagus and cheese.

PAULA'S OKRA GUMBO

3 T organic olive oil

3 T whole wheat flour

1 organic green pepper, chopped

1-2 organic celery stalks, chopped

1 organic yellow onion, chopped

1 15 or 16-ounce can organic stewed tomatoes

or 2 C fresh organic chopped tomatoes

1 C organic vegetable or chicken broth

2 C organic okra, sliced into ¼-inch-thick rounds

1 T Worcestershire sauce

1 T Tabasco or other Louisiana-style hot sauce

¾ t sea salt

½ t organic black pepper

½ t organic dried thyme

1 C filtered water

3 C organic basmati or brown rice, cooked

In a stockpot, heat oil over medium heat and stir in flour. Cook, stirring constantly, until the flour is browned but not burned, about 10 minutes. Add green pepper, celery and onion and cook over medium heat until just tender. Stir in tomatoes, broth, okra, Worcestershire sauce, hot sauce, salt, pepper, thyme and water, bring to a boil. Reduce heat and simmer 20–25 minutes to blend the flavors. Serve with the cooked rice.

GARLIC SWEET POTATOES

4 medium organic sweet potatoes, cut lengthwise into thick wedges

1 t sea salt

¼ t organic black pepper

¼ C organic olive oil, *divided use*

4 organic garlic cloves, finely chopped and from the USA, not China

Preheat oven to 450 degrees. Place potatoes on a baking sheet and toss with salt, pepper and 3 T of the olive oil. Roast until potatoes are browned, 30–35 minutes, turning them over once, halfway through, to brown evenly. Combine garlic and remaining oil in a bowl. Brush potatoes with garlic and oil mixture. Roast until garlic is cooked, 2–4 minutes.

KOHLRABI STIR-FRY
½ organic onion, sliced
2 T unsalted organic butter, *divided use*
2 C kohlrabi, cut into ½-inch chunks
½ C sliced baby bella mushrooms
1 ½ T oyster sauce
2 T chopped parsley
10- to 12-ounce broiled lean sirloin steak, cut into thin strips (free-range and antibiotic and hormone free)
2 C cooked angel hair pasta
Sea salt
Organic black pepper

Cook onion in skillet with 1 T butter for 2–3 minutes over medium heat. Add kohlrabi, mushrooms, oyster sauce, parsley and remaining butter and cook over medium heat 5–7 minutes. Add steak and cooked pasta to skillet. Continue cooking, tossing until meat is heated through. Season with salt and pepper.

ROASTED BRUSSELS SPROUTS
2 pounds Brussels sprouts, halved lengthwise
¼ C organic olive oil
¼ t sea salt
¼ t organic black pepper
1 t organic dried thyme

1 t organic garlic, chopped and from the USA, not China
Cooking spray
1/3 C grated Parmesan

Preheat oven to 450 degrees. Place sprouts in large mixing bowl. Add oil, salt, pepper, thyme, garlic and mix to coat. Lightly spray a baking sheet with cooking spray. Place sprouts in single layer on baking sheet and roast in heated oven 10–15 minutes. To cook evenly, carefully turn sprouts over halfway through. Add Parmesan. Roast another 10 minutes and check to see whether sprouts are evenly browned. When browned and cheese melted, serve in a bowl.

SMOKY PEAS AND POTATOES
1½ pounds small organic new or red potatoes
1½ pounds fresh peas (1½ C shelled, or use organic frozen peas)
2 T unsalted organic butter
2 T whole wheat flour
1⅔ C raw organic milk
6 ounces raw milk smoked cheese
4 slices smoked bacon (free-range and antibiotic-free pork) cooked and crumbled, *divided use*

Cook potatoes in boiling water until done, 15–20 minutes. Drain. Cook peas in small amount of boiling water until tender, 8–15 minutes. In a small saucepan, melt butter, stir in flour and add milk. Cook, stirring until mixture thickens and bubbles. Cut cheese into small pieces and add to sauce. Cook and stir over low heat, adding ½ the crumbled bacon to sauce. Combine potatoes and peas in a dish, pour cheese sauce over and finish with other ½ of crumbled bacon.

ORGANIC COCONUT MACAROONS
½ c unsalted organic butter, softened
1 C organic coconut palm sugar
4 eggs (free-range)
1 t organic vanilla
1 t organic raw chia seeds
¼ t organic cinnamon
½ C organic coconut flour
2 C organic shredded unsweetened coconut
Organic coconut oil

Preheat oven to 375 degrees. Mix together butter, sugar, eggs, vanilla, chia seeds and cinnamon. Stir in coconut flour and coconut; mix well. Grease a baking sheet with the coconut oil. Drop tablespoon-size mounds, about 2 inches apart, onto baking sheet. Bake 12–15 minutes until golden brown. Remove from baking sheet and cool on wire rack. Makes about 24 cookies.

APPLE CRISP
4 organic apples, peeled and thinly sliced
½ C organic coconut palm sugar
½ C whole wheat flour
½ C organic oats
¾ t organic cinnamon
¾ t organic nutmeg
6 T organic unsalted butter

Preheat oven to 375 degrees. Lightly grease sides of a large pie plate. Arrange apple slices on plate. Mix remaining ingredients in a bowl. Sprinkle mixture over apples. Bake about 40 minutes or until topping is golden brown and apples are tender.

Chapter 13   Acupuncture

First, I meet with Ericka, the office assistant at Dr. Steuber's office. I give her the history of the past six months.

Dr. Steuber comes in and impresses me again. He's very knowledgeable and says, "I've worked with cancer patients before."

I rely on my intuition a lot lately and I get a good feeling here.

Jack and I each take a test on a pulse machine. You hold on to metal bars, your body gets scanned and a printout tells how balanced you are. I did better than Jack, which makes me nervous. Jack does so much for me: the new vegan diet, the juices two times a day, the oxy aloe, the E3Live. He takes me to every doctor appointment. I want Jack to have some treatments.

"Jack, maybe you should get some treatments, too?" I suggest.

"No, let Dr. Steuber take care of you first."

He won't agree to any treatments.

The doctor explains: "Your body has meridians that carry energy. Stimulation of specific acupuncture points, by needling, improves energy and balance, which can result in stimulation of the body's natural healing abilities."

Exactly what I like to hear.

I see Dr. Steuber twice a week. Each treatment room is large enough to fit an acupuncture table, a chair to put your pocketbook on and a small chest of drawers holding supplies. There's soft music playing.

Dr. Steuber says, "Something traumatic had to have happened to let the cancer manifest in your body. You wear your emotions on the top of your skin and you have to lift the veils so we can get to the problem."

He places needles in the fleshy part of the skin between my thumb and pointer finger, in several places on my ears, and in four different areas of my feet. The needles are placed at meridian points that connect with my colon— also at points that are to help me let go.

I lie still for 30 to 35 minutes to let the process take effect.

I listen to the music and pray the Rosary. I think about what could have happened to me that was traumatic?

Perhaps it was that I lost my mother to cancer and within a couple of months lost two businesses due to the poor economy. But I thought I'd handled those situations fine.

At a self-help course, though, I learned that the acronym *FINE* means *f**ked-up, insecure, neurotic and empty.*

Oh, well, I'll lift those veils because I have to get better.

In June, I have ten doctor appointments, along with weddings, Father's Day picnics, trips to the mountains and our eighteenth wedding anniversary. Only eight doctor appointments in July. Summer is flying by.

Chapter 14   Grace

Jack set up a one-on-one meeting with Grace Asagra, a business associate from his Networking & More group. Grace is a holistic nurse and integrative health coach.

We bumped into her in the hospital lobby toward the end of my radiation. I want to meet for coffee to make sure our personalities work well together. My hope is that she can help me stay on track with my diet. Ironically, our first meeting is at the café in Whole Foods.

Grace is a beautiful, petite Filipino. Her features are truly exotic and she has a bronze skin tone and inquisitive, yet friendly, eyes and shiny black hair that cascades down the middle of her back.

I like Grace from the get-go. She's easy to talk to, understanding and has amazing energy.

She tells me her story: "Before starting my own private practice, I was a critical care nurse in a conventional hospital for twenty years."

"Why did you leave such a great job?" I wonder.

"I can no longer continue to support medical treatments I don't believe in."

Grace's business card is impressive. She has Certification in Holistic Nursing and Certification in Critical Care Nursing. She is a registered nurse and has a Master of Arts and Science. She's also Certified in Neuroscience and Certified in Integrative Nutrition.

I tell her, "I think it takes a lot of courage to sacrifice a good steady corporate income and face business uncertainties for the love of empowering people to control their health care."

I tell her my story and I'm happy to hear Grace also believes that the body can heal itself naturally.

"In my practice, I've observed what indigenous healers have taught us all along— that for every illness, there is an underlying emotion as well as a pattern of behavior long before one gets diagnosed," she says.

I reply: "Right now, I'm working on fear issues and – more importantly – anger issues. A lot of people irritate me. I also let world situations get to me."

She says: "You do have to be careful. In my experience, all negative emotions feed illness. It's important to contemplate and notice your ways in the past, but, most importantly your ways in the present."

We decide on monthly phone conversations. Grace also e-mails me diet suggestions.

This month, we talk about diet changes.

"Paula, you don't want to feed the cancer, so I'd like you to stay away from sugar, gluten and dairy. And for now, no meat."

"What am I supposed to eat? I love yogurt, grains and meat."

"You can still have grains except for wheat, barley, rye and buckwheat. You still have lots of choices. You can have fruits, vegetables and legumes. You can have one portion of whole grains, like brown rice or quinoa daily. If you must, you can have one dairy daily. I'll e-mail you a selection of menus that will be favorable for you."

One grain a day is going to be hard. I love grains. This diet is overwhelming, but I'll do my best.

"You have to eat to live, not live to eat." Grace says.

Later, I tell Jack, "I'm not sure this health-coaching thing is working out."

"I thought everything was going fine. You're doing great."

"Well, it's not going fine. Every time I get used to a food item that Grace asks me to eliminate, she asks me to eliminate yet another item. I'm not a happy camper. I'm not even fun to be around anymore. This detoxing is like withdrawal."

Being the perfect cheerleader, Jack says: "Paula, hang in there, you're doing so well. It's going to get easier. I promise."

In our conversation today, Grace is getting to know the good, the bad and the ugly sides of me. After spending hours on the phone with an insurance company, I rant about how incompetent and apathetic people are about their jobs, only I don't say it that nicely, I say, "I can't stand people and I really can't stand stupid people!"

In a calm voice, Grace asks: "How are your relationships? How about with your mother? Your father? Your sisters? Jack? Your daughter? Others? I am asking these questions because often we look too far for sources of problems, when many times we may have issues from the past that we hold on to, instead of forgiving them. We can't beat ourselves on and on and over and over. If we do that to ourselves, how then would others treat us? Your anger is not going to help you. Colon cancer is about letting go. Let go of the stories of the past that do not help you. Ask yourself questions like: Do I feel good about these feelings? Are they serving any purpose? Does it make sense? Does it solve the problem?"

I tell her: "I'm definitely working on forgiveness. I know I over-react sometimes. I'm working on that too." I think to myself, *nothing a JoJo's pizza and a pitcher of Yuengling wouldn't cure.*

My homework assignment this month is to be more agreeable—like Jack is! He's always agreeable and it's being brought to my attention that—I'm *not*!

No matter who I talk to, the main message that keeps coming through loud and clear is: Learn how to let go.

Life is stressful. I'm working hard to acquire tools in my toolbox to keep my stress levels in check.

Stress happens and I have to learn to deal with it.

I guess I'm a work in progress.

Grace tells me: "Your body holds on to emotions-- particularly negative emotions. Eventually, those emotions become physical symptoms. Negative emotions are stored mostly in fat cells. Our body loves us so much that it will continue to make adjustments for us, but eventually, the emotions may manifest in some form of cancer or auto-immune disease or chronic condition that just won't leave us until we change our behaviors."

Food, as medicine, has always played a big part in our work together. Today, Grace is teaching me about the value of fermented foods.

It's funny: when my sisters tried to tell me about the benefits of raw milk, raw yogurt and fermented foods like kombucha, I didn't listen.

Kombucha is a fermented probiotic drink that originated in China. It's now available in any grocery store. My sisters make it themselves from tea, sugar, a SCOBY and a starter from the previous batch.

SCOBY is an acronym for *symbiotic colony* of *bacteria* and *yeast*. In short, it consists of beneficial bacteria and yeast that work together to produce a certain type of fermented culture. Kombucha is fermented over a course of 7-31 days. The final product is naturally carbonated, making this a fizzy and tasty drink.

It also has amazing health benefits, like improved digestion and detoxification of the liver, and it's high in antioxidants that destroy free-radicals, which can cause cancer.

I don't know why we don't listen to family, but when Grace suggests it, I'm all for it.

This is a whole new ball game. My diet has changed radically.

Grace teaches me, "You should have at least a tablespoon of fermented food with every meal – particularly fermented vegetables like kimchi."

"Kimchi?"

"Kimchi is a traditional Korean fermented side dish made with vegetables and a variety of seasonings, usually pickled cabbage. All ancient cultures around the world practice fermentation, a process that preserves food and creates beneficial enzymes, B-vitamins, omega-3 fatty acids and various strains of probiotics. Fermented foods pre-digest carbohydrates so we don't put a heavy load on our digestive system.

Fermented foods support nutrients necessary for the body. This is crucial because the whole body has trillions more bacteria cells than human cells. Although the microbiome is all over the body, the highest concentration and largest diversity are in the gastrointestinal tract.

Gut health is maintained when the microbiota in our digestive system are well balanced. When gut health is in homeostasis, the rest of the body moves toward healing and recovery. Fermented foods help balance microbiota."

"Sauerkraut and pickles are fermented; will they qualify?" I ask.

"Correct they qualify."

"I thought I ate healthier than most Americans when all of this started, but I'm learning so much about food from you, Grace. Thank you."

Between the chemo, the radiation and the diet change, I didn't understand why the weight hadn't been falling off me. Working with Grace has produced the best results. I lose twelve pounds in two months.

"I want us to start doing Hilot, the healing massage I learned when I was growing up in the Philippines," Grace says. "Hilot is first aid in my culture and our immediate go-to intervention when we're not feeling well."

"Hilot? What does it mean?" I asked.

"The word *hilot* refers to the healing ways, such as massage, herbs and rituals that heal. A manghihilot is the person doing the healing. I find it hard to explain to those not immersed in the culture. It simply means healing is about to take place when you use hilot. It's not so much about the person doing the healing, but the intention and the intervention that the healer provides for the patient. In hilot, we recognize and respect the presence of positive energy that surrounds us. With that positive energy, we work on disharmony that's not just in the body, but also in the mind, heart and spirit."

Grace also introduces me to Qigong.

"I think Qigong is the perfect energy work for you to incorporate into your daily practice. It uses slow motions to generate the energy that surrounds you. It's good for your physical body, your mental body and your emotional body. *Qi* means *breath* and *gong* means *discipline*. We'll work on the basics at our next meeting."

I see Grace once a month for healing massages now. Her massages are amazing and more therapeutic. As a registered nurse, Grace knows every part of the human body. Growing up in the Philippines, she learned to incorporate the art of Asian healing, which makes this massage like none I've ever experienced. When we're done, I feel as if I'm floating on a cloud.

Through very personal conversations about letting go of fear, forgiving past hurts and accepting whatever happens in the future, coupled with the massages, creates a calmness in me.

Incorporating positive affirmation is also included in my daily practice. Grace teaches me to say, "I am enough, I have enough, and I do enough."

Because of Grace, Jack and I are practicing yoga again. We also meditate more.

Grace emphasizes: "There are many research articles proving that meditation is important to achieve health, contentment and long life. It is good to practice sitting meditation regularly at least fifteen minutes and then longer. Meditation can take place even while you're working, driving, eating or doing daily chores. For every breath you take, there is an opportunity to experience openness and spaciousness."

I can't say enough about Grace. She is generous with her love, her joy and her wisdom. She's interested in everyone and sends out positive energy. Her caring comes straight from her heart. Grace is beautiful inside and out.

I am the luckiest person to have had God put Grace in my path.

Grace has also written a book about massage called *The Healing Dance: A Fusion of Massage and Asian Healing Arts*.

Chapter 15   Compounded Hormones

I see Dr. Bartiss on Tuesdays and Thursdays. I love him; he's so excited about helping me get rid of this cancer. He orders an extensive blood test. I join the Life Extension organization so that I can get the test for only $400. It usually costs $2,400.

Mark also has purchased a new ozone sauna machine, which opens the pores. The ozone goes into the machine and then goes directly into the pores.

Wow. It's a lot cheaper, too. I want Jack to try it.

It's September 20, 2012, and no matter what, I plan on having a happy birthday. I start the day with a 10 a.m. appointment at Dr. Bartiss'.

I tell him: "I have slight cramping in my pelvic area. I'm eliminating clear mucus and, yesterday, I saw a drop of blood. Besides, that change in my BM habit, I feel great."

He tells me, "Don't worry about the clear mucus or the drop of blood. If blood is there every day, then yes, worry. One drop, don't worry."

Today I do the ozone sauna for the first time.

Mark instructs us on how to use the sauna. The fiberglass sauna closet opens to expose an adjustable seat. I strip naked, put towels on the seat so my rear can be comfortable, then Jack closes the doors, with just my head sticking out.

There's no room to move. I feel as if I'm in a small capsule. Towels are then placed around the opening and around my neck so the ozone can't escape into the room.

To lighten the situation, Jack says, "This looks like a scene from 'I Love Lucy'"

Only I'm not laughing. "It looks like a sauna from a 1950s gym to me, Ricky."

The idea is for my pores to open from the heat so that the ozone can go directly into my body through the open pores.

This will oxygenate the blood. Cancer cannot live in oxygenated blood.

"Oh, my God, 108 degrees is HOT HOT HOT!"

I'm to stay in the sauna for half an hour. Jack makes business calls and I watch TV to try to make the time go by faster.

It's not working.

I'm so hot and my hands are inside the capsule, so Jack has to wipe away the sweat that is dripping off of my heat flushed face.

I feel claustrophobic.

"Jack, get me out of here!"

I lasted only eighteen minutes.

Mark wants me to do the sauna every time I come for an ultraviolet treatment.

Next Monday, he also wants to make an incision in the upper layer of skin on my butt in order to insert hormone pellets.

I want more info about what's involved with this before I do it. For instance, how long do they last and how much do they cost?

After a couple of business appointments, Jack and I meet Lois and my friend, Dassy, for a birthday lunch at home. Lois brings fresh veggies and fruit. Dassy brings a bottle of organic wine, chocolate cupcakes and a beautiful yellow mum.

Another friend leaves a present on the front porch and I receive more than a hundred birthday wishes on Facebook. My brother calls, my nieces text a birthday song and the card from my daughter, Katie, is so thoughtful, it makes me cry.

I'm a lucky, happy girl. Oh, and Susan's coming to the mountains this weekend to pamper me.

Lois tells me, "Suzanne Somers has a new cable TV show that airs at 7 a.m. once a week on Mondays."

"Great! I'll DVR it so I don't miss any shows," I tell her.

"I'm not sure how long the show will last because she's allowing only advertisers that comply with healthy lifestyles. So, there will be no pharmaceutical commercials or any food products like those from General Mills, Campbell's or Nabisco because they use genetically engineered ingredients.

I say, "Good for her: I like that she's standing by her principles."

Lois continues: "I was also reading about the top ten genetically modified foods. Corn is at the top of the list and high-fructose corn syrup is in almost everything."

"What else was on the list?" I ask.

"Sugar, soy, canola, dairy and zucchini are what I remember off the top of my head. They have strict laws against GMOs in Europe. Most Americans don't even know what GMOs are."

"I know, and it's not as if you can just be a good label reader, because our government is fighting to stop GMO labeling." I say.

"OK, I'll bite," Dassy chimes in. "What exactly is a GMO?"

"Lois, can you take this question please."

Lois explains: "GMOs, or genetically modified organisms, are living organisms whose genetic material has been artificially manipulated in a laboratory through genetic engineering. It's a process in which genes from the DNA of one species get extracted and then get artificially forced into the genes of an unrelated plant or animal. The foreign genes may come from viruses, insects, animals or even humans."

"Oh, boy, you got her started," I chuckle. "It's a controversial subject. For some people, the jury is still out on whether there are health risks associated with GMOs."

Lois says, "I believe there are."

I can't believe it! Suzanne Somers's first show is about compounded-hormone replacement therapy and how it changed her life.

Is God sending me messages on cable TV?

Somers says, "Hormones are to the human body as water is to a plant. Without water the plant dries up."

OK, water is important.

When I meet with Dr. Bartiss again, he tells me: "Compounded hormones are different from synthetic ones. The compounded hormones are created specifically for you."

"Bioidentical compounded hormones boost the immune system and help keep cancer away from the breasts, cervix, colon and bladder."

After hearing that, I let Mark insert the hormone pellets.

He also orders from a compound pharmacy certain progesterone and thyroid hormones in capsule form that will be mailed directly to me by tomorrow.

Chapter 16   The Holy Spirit

A big storm is coming and Jack and I are at Eagle Lake in the mountains.

They're calling it Frankenstorm.

The media has succeeded at panicking everyone, so we leave early. I'm glad we're home. They now call the storm Sandy. We have family and friends who own homes in the storm's path.

I love Halloween.

Jack doesn't.

We have three masquerade parties to go to. One's being hosted by our dance instructor; one's for the Stray Cats organization and, finally, there's a house party.

I'm a Viking warrior princess and Jack's a cook. My headdress is a bejeweled, horned helmet with different colored stones and long blonde braided pigtails attached. I finish the outfit with a tattered Viking gown. Jack's costume consists of a puffy chef hat and an apron he uses at home.

Even though we don't match, we win the people's choice award at the dance party.

Jack really knows how to *spice it up* on the dance floor.

By the time, we get to the house party, Jack doesn't even have his chef hat on.

Hurricane Sandy is touted the second-most costly storm in US history. They say it was the deadliest and most destructive hurricane of 2012. There were 115-mile-per-hour winds and $68 billion in damage.

Speaking of storms, after Halloween I always feel as if the next two months fly by. Because the cancer diagnosis was around the Christmas and New Year's holidays, I want to have a colonoscopy before this year's holidays.

Dr. Logan says, "A sigmoidoscopy and an ultrasound with pictures will suffice for now."

So mid-November, I make another trip to the hospital.

Right when we see the pictures, Jack and I just grin at each other.

We're excited because to the naked eye, it looks as if the tumor has shrunk — a lot.

It looks like nothing more than smooth scar tissue against the colon wall.

Dr. Logan doesn't even recognize that it is obviously much smaller and says, "You have a polyp that could be a problem."

I ask, "Why didn't you remove it?"

She replies, "It will be taken care of when we operate."

Yeah, I don't think so. It's been almost six months since the last pictures and the tumor is now flush against the wall of the colon. This is amazing! I'm going to continue what I'm doing, for it is obviously working.

My high school friend, Debbie, tells me: "My sister Cindy boards her horse at Pat's stables. Pat is especially spiritual and has personally experienced faith-filled healings in her own family."

Pat invites us to meet her at her church, New Hope Church of God in East Windsor.

We drive along a country road and come to an intersection with corn fields to the right and pastures to the left. There stands a building that looks like it's from a different century.

It's a small white church with a tall steeple.

Debbie, Cindy, Jack and I arrive at the church before Pat. The congregation is very welcoming.

We're greeted at the front door by a woman named Ruby, who is dressed to perfection.

"Are you Pat's friends?" she asks.

A little surprised, we say, "Yes."

"She told us you were coming and we're gonna take good care of y'all. Now come with me."

She escorts us into the church, which has no more than fifteen rows of wooden pews. Ruby wants us to sit in the middle of the church, row 7 or 8. She makes some regular parishioners move so that we could all sit in the same pew and save a spot for Pat.

It's a tight-knit church. Everyone here can tell we're new.

It's Pentecostal and there is a lot of singing, amen, and hallelujahs. There's hand clapping, people waving things in the air and swaying back and forth.

I see Cindy greet someone who squeezes in at the end of our pew.

It must be Pat.

Debbie and I giggle and she says, "This isn't the way we did it at Notre Dame."

"I'm really enjoying it," I tell her.

"Me too," she says.

Pat gets my attention by waving to me and smiling. She also sends a note down the aisle that says, "Don't be afraid. John 3:16."

The pastor appears at the back of the church.

While gospel music plays, the pastor struts down the aisle and everyone is going wild. He's wearing a teal blue suit that fits him perfectly. His wife is already at the altar, sitting in a place of honor. She, too, is dressed to the nines. The organist is on the altar pounding away on the organ and everyone is praising God.

Everybody, including our group, is clapping hands and dancing. It's like the church scene with James Brown in the Blues Brothers movie.

I try to give Jack something to wave in the air, but he looks at me as if to say, *Where have you taken me now?*

He says, "If I want to wave something in the air, I'll find it myself, thanks."

This is like nothing I've ever experienced before.

I can't wipe the smile off my face.

I hope everyone in my group is OK with how long we're here.

It started at 10:30. It's now 12:30 and it doesn't look like the service is ending anytime soon.

At one point, the pastor asks, "Who wants to come up to the altar and be prayed over?"

Pat wiggles past everyone in the aisle to get to me and encourages me to go to the altar. In fact, she grabs my hand and takes me there herself.

She hands me over to Elder Jerome, who asks me, "What would you be praying for today?"

I whisper, "For God to remove the cancer from my body."

Oh, my God, did Elder Jerome give that cancer a talking to.

He's quoting all sorts of Bible passages about healing and saying, "All you have to do is believe! All things are possible through Christ!" and "God, You take the cancer cells out of Paula's body right NOW!"

He's screaming in my ear.

Oh yeah! I believe!

The room is emotionally charged.

I hold tightly to his hands.

I'm getting weak in the knees.

I feel a hand on my back and I hold on to it.

I'm telling you, he wants me to fall to the ground.

I end up sitting down in the first pew that's behind me.

Jack comes over and holds me.

It's wild.

The whole church is praising God.

You can feel the Holy Spirit.

Something extremely powerful is going on.

We're there ever so long and everyone's getting hungry. I can hardly believe the congregation sent us home with full chicken dinners—veggies and dessert and everything. All of it homemade by church members.

After the service, we all go to Pat's horse farm to eat the chicken and discuss the experience we'd just had.

Pat's Bible was opened to John 3:16, which reads, "For God so loved the world, that he gave his only begotten Son, that whosoever believeth in him should not perish, but have everlasting life."

Everything is delicious.

We all agree that something powerful had happened that day at the New Hope Church of God.

Chapter 17   Cancer Is Big Business

It's mid-February. January had been tough on my veins. It's no longer easy to get blood from the one spot where blood used to flow easily. My honey spot has run dry.

"I'm going to Florida for two weeks. Why don't you take a break from Dr. Bartiss' office while I'm gone," says the technician who administers the intravenous treatments.

"No problem, I can use the break, too. See you in March."

I take daily supplements—twelve pills in the morning, twelve in the evening. One of them Lois found while doing her cancer research is called vitamin B_{17}, or amygdalin or laetrile. Laetrile is known to shrink tumors. The greatest concentration of laetrile is found in apricot pits and bitter nuts like almonds.

It's hard to find, though, because several years ago, vitamin B_{17} was banned from sale in the United States.

I ask myself, *Why?*

Apparently, it contains trace amounts of cyanide.

Well, because chemotherapy poisons the body and radiation burns it, *shouldn't I be allowed to choose my own poison?*

Jack finds a company in Mexico that sells laetrile online. I add it to my daily supplement intake.

In the news, recently, two young girls were taken away from their parents so that the state can give them medical treatments the government deems is best for those kids.

I wonder whether someday the conventional doctors will be able to force me to have an operation I don't believe will cure me.

After all, it's what they feel is in my best interest.

One doctor did suggest I need psychological help.

Talk about scary.

Could doctors say I'm not well enough to make good decisions for myself?

One girl named Cassandra C, from Connecticut is forced to undergo chemotherapy even though she doesn't want to. Cassandra wants to seek alternative treatments first. She is seventeen years old and her mother stands by her decision.

The state of Connecticut takes this child away from her mother. The mother lawyers up, but the Connecticut Supreme Court judge rules that the daughter must remain at the Connecticut Children's Medical Center in Hartford under temporary custody of the state Department of Children and Families until she completes her court-ordered chemotherapy.

Why have this young woman's and her mother's rights been taken away?

Then there's the story about the doctor in Detroit. Dr. Farid Fata, who defrauded Medicare by telling people they had cancer so he could give them chemotherapy treatments and be reimbursed.

Cancer is a lucrative business and this doctor fraudulently recouped seventeen million dollars just by prescribing cancer treatments even though 553 cancer-free patients received medically unnecessary infusions or injections.

Cancer is big business—so big there's a school of thought that says big pharma doesn't want to find a cure for cancer.

Or, if they've already found a cure, they're keeping it hidden from the public.

One of the doctors associated with my conventional cancer team challenges me to find clinical trials that prove that change of diet would have a positive effect.

When I looked for studies, I found evidence of clinical trials started, but then sabotaged by lack of funding. Pharmaceutical companies—even though they get money from the government – won't fund those studies because doing so wouldn't fit into their business plans. In fact, it threatens their profit centers.

I'm so excited to see Kelly Turner, a researcher, publish a book recounting the stories of a thousand people she interviewed who healed themselves naturally. The book is called *Radical Remission*. The author says that all of those interviewed radically changed their diets and lived to tell about it.

In my research, I came across a documentary on Dr. Stanislaw Burzynski, who runs a clinic in Houston. His cancer work is especially beneficial for brain cancers in children and the doctor has also been successful with several other types of cancers.

His protocol is called anti-neoplaston therapy, which consists of the use of a non-toxic, gene-targeted medicine with no side effects like those from chemo and radiation. The treatment turns off oncogenes that cause cancer and it activates tumor suppressor genes.

The documentary describes harassment of the doctor that began in the 1970's by big medicine, big pharma, the Food and Drug Administration (FDA), National Cancer Institute and the Texas Medical Board.

Evidence shows that the US FDA pressured the Texas Medical Board to revoke Burzynski's medical license—despite the fact that he had broken no laws and his treatment was proved safe and effective.

But those large institutions were relentless and they continued to pursue Dr. Burzynski by taking him to a higher court and ultimately to the Texas Supreme Court. Even though the organization knew the treatments worked, the FDA said the treatments had never been approved by the agency.

They even tried to put him in prison for life.

The government agencies always lost their cases.

The Burzynski Clinic is the clinic where Thomas Navarro's parents wanted him to go that led to introduction of the Thomas Navarro FDA Patient Rights Act (H.R. 3677) in Congress.

For eighteen months, the FDA prohibited Thomas from treatment at the Burzynski Clinic. Only when Thomas was declared terminally ill and given only fourteen days to live did the FDA allow him to go to the Houston clinic. By that time, though, it was too late because the complications caused by the chemotherapy had made it impossible to save the child's life.

Why would these powerful institutions continue to try to stop Dr. Burzynski's clinic from helping cancer patients?

The medical establishment is composed of universities, professional organizations, published journals, regulatory agencies, researchers, scientists, funding agencies and countless individuals – all of them with differing incentives and perspectives. The idea that they would all be in on a massive conspiracy to hide perhaps the greatest cure known to mankind is beyond absurd.

Or is it?

What I've found in the past couple of years is that *prevention* is the "cure" for cancer.

Clean up what you eat.

Try eating only genetically-modified-organism-free and pesticide-free food.

We do have to pay extra for organic food even though that's the kind of food most of us grew up on. It's only during the past twenty or thirty years that Monsanto messed with our food supply by filling the fields with pesticides like Roundup.

According to the Centers for Disease Control and Prevention, 1.66 million new cancer cases were diagnosed in 2013.

In the 1940's, only one in sixteen people developed cancer.

In the 1970's, it was one in ten.

Today it's one in three!

There has been a war on cancer for forty years. Why are one in three of us going to experience it?

I think it has something to do with diet and the immune system. Once you detoxify your body from toxic food in order to keep your immune system healthy, the rest of the healing is spiritual, emotional and mental.

Ultimately, no matter what treatment you choose to try to cure your cancer, it's your immune system that's doing all the hard work.

All I know is, every time I get checked, the cancer markers are lower and the tumor is disappearing.

I've had a busy and exciting year of following all the new techniques I've learned.

The months are flying by and its already September. My weight is stable. I do ozone treatments three times a week at home and I see Dr. Bartiss once a month. I'm also due for hormone pellets.

I feel a little anxious because I just made an appointment with Dr. Logan for October 7. I want to take a peek at whether the tumor is still shrinking. I don't know why I'm so nervous; all the good things I do for my body surely have to be helping. I relax more. I'm learning to let go more. I pray a lot and I know my body can heal itself.

I feel great and I feel healthy.

My appointment with Dr. Logan is at 10am today. Linda, the attending nurse, is very calming and compassionate.

I'm surprised Dr. Logan wants to take a look with a sigmoidoscopy.

She also does a digital exam.

I ask, "Do you feel anything?"

Not answering my question, she says, "Let me try the scope again."

She uses the scope again and I ask again, "Can you see anything?"

She says she cannot see anything, but adds, "We'll set up a colonoscopy to see what's happening."

I have to ask a third time whether she feels anything before she admits, "I feel something hard."

I'm thinking it could be scar tissue.

She orders an ultrasound with biopsies and a colonic polypectomy.

Dr. Logan is still not as optimistic as I am about the tumor's shrinkage.

When I suggest, "The ultrasound may show how much the tumor has shrunk and may even show the tumor is no longer in the wall of the colon."

Dr. Logan just says, "That's not likely."

I get extremely excited once I leave the exam. I realize that if she saw it or felt anything significant, she would have said, "Whoop, there it is!"

I'm concerned about the biopsies. I like the strategy of touch me not—or leave it alone.

Even if the cancer's still there, it's not going to change my course of treatment.

But I don't want to give Dr. Logan any ammunition so she can say, "See, it's still there, so let me cut it out."

I believe in miracles. I believe the body can heal itself.

I have an appointment on October 14 for a colonoscopy and an ultrasound.

First, they want blood work done, an EKG and a chest X-ray. A CAT scan will be done after the colonoscopy.

Linda, the nurse, schedules all the tests and even sets up a follow-up appointment to go over the results on Monday, October 21 at 9:45 a.m.

Chapter 18   What's It Gonna Be?

Jack and I are sitting in the waiting room feeling tense because Dr. Logan will give us the test results of the biopsies, ultrasound and CAT scan. I look anxiously at my cell phone. 9:45. This may be a blue Monday or a light one. I note the date: October 21, 2013 and I pray my guardian angels are close by.

It's so quiet I can hear the second hand of the wall clock ticking as it inches slowly through its cycle.

"Paula Beiger?" the receptionist calls out.

"I'm here," I respond and she escorts us to the examining room.

We're now waiting in the smaller room — the one where you see the doctor. The room is very plain with white cabinets. On the wall are a rubber glove dispenser and a poster of the human body with the organs exposed. There's one patient table with white disposable paper on it and two nondescript chairs.

We sit there quietly. Again, I realize how lucky I am because no matter what the outcome, Jack is with me and he will continue to support me, love me and make this rocky road as smooth as possible. It's easy to be strong when you have that kind of attention.

Dr. Logan enters the room with no emotion whatsoever. Her hair is in a neat and tight ponytail. She has on a white coat with two big pockets in the front and stylish but sensible shoes.

With clipboard in hand, she says, "Let's get right to it." She starts summarizing from the top of my stomach and works her way down.

"First, the CAT scan shows lung nodules all clear. Lymph nodes clear also. Stomach clear."

But there's a small lesion on my liver. It was there two years ago and is now smaller. Not a problem.

"Intestines clear."

Everything so far is clear, yet no smiles from Dr. Logan.

"Now, for the eight biopsies." She says stoically. "Upper colon no malignancy and a polyp was taken out. Mid colon no malignancy. Lower colon benign, but there's a polyp forming. Descending colon no malignancy."

OK, we're now down to where the tumor is and Jack and I are waiting for a shoe to drop. I sit tensely on the patient table with my hands stiffly holding on to either side. Jack is sitting to the right of me and Dr. Logan on my left.

"With biopsies done all around and right into the tumor—all are benign. No malignancy."

I say, "Are you telling me there is no cancer?

"That's right: no cancer."

Oh, my God. I can hardly believe it, even though this is what I believed all along would happen.

NO CANCER!

I immediately change, in my mind, the word *unbelievable* to the word *amazing*!

Even with the amazing news of no cancer found, Dr. Logan cannot smile. In fact, she sucks the joy right out of the room. She doesn't even give Jack and me a chance to celebrate, hug, kiss or jump for joy!

She immediately adds, "The only recommendation is that you still have surgery"—which would consist of removal of my rectum, removal of part of my colon and insertion of a permanent colostomy bag.

Jack and I have only a moment to smile at each other. The news hasn't really sunk in.

Without any discussion, Dr. Logan knows she can't sell me on the surgery.

I didn't want surgery when cancer was present and I certainly won't agree to it with *no* cancer present.

I ask, "What would be your plan B, because surgery is obviously not my first choice?"

Dr. Logan replies: "I have no plan B for you. My one and only recommendation is surgery. Other countries with patients in your situation may follow up and keep checking to make sure nothing grows, but here in the United States the standard of practice consists of chemotherapy, radiation and surgery."

Why would anyone in their right mind do this surgery without having to?

She also tells us of an eighty-two-year-old woman whom she is to operate on later this week. The woman has a similar growth yet has never had any cancer.
"The patient chose to have the operation that I'm recommending so as to avoid the cancer's ever happening."
Are you kidding me? Talking an eighty-two-year-old into having a life-changing operation — or should I say, scaring her into it — equals malpractice in my book.
I hope she doesn't think that telling me such a story is going to change my opinion about surgery.
Dr. Logan adds, "I feel you're looking for my approval for your course of action." — or lack of action in the form of no surgery.
I was not looking for approval and I told her so. "I respect *your* knowledge and opinion. All I want in return is *your* respect for *my* opinion. After all, it is my body."
She then asks, "What do you think you're teaching your daughter?"
I say, "I hope I'm teaching her to think for herself."

Because she will not give me a plan B, Dr. Logan doesn't even recommend my coming in for a three, six, or twelve-month checkup and/or colonoscopy.

I tell her, "I have my own cancer support group of friends who have lived with and survived cancer. I will ask them what their doctors have recommended."

She then orders an MRI because she's still looking for something medically wrong with me.

She also recommends that I see my oncologist.

Then I am curtly dismissed.

She doesn't know how to deal with a patient who doesn't go along with her recommendation.

Jack finishes up paperwork at the reception area.

Back in the waiting room, I look up at the ceiling and run my fingers through my hair. I say to myself, *This is really happening! I am really cancer free!* I think I may have even said it aloud. I don't care what the other people in the room think of my talking to myself. I just received news I'm having trouble processing.

I'm in my own little world and feel almost numb. I don't know how to react to the recent information. Don't understand why the doctor didn't burst into the room, all smiles and excited, to tell me the wonderful news that I was now cancer free!

Instead, she made such great news actually uncomfortable.

But the moment Jack and I leave the office, feelings of joy start to flood every cell in my body. I'm ready to explode with happiness. I want to jump up and down like a little kid on a playground. As we walk to the car, we look at each other. I shake my head. I don't know what to say. I have trouble expressing myself. All I know is that everything is different now.

Jack, with a smile beaming on his face, says, "We did it!"

We didn't expect this news today, so we have a calendar full of business appointments.

We begin calling friends with the news.

Chapter 19   Pure Joy

Our first appointment is in New Hope, Pennsylvania. While we're on our way, I start calling the twelve people who know I have cancer. I call Katie, my sisters, my brother and all those who supported me in the past two years. With each call I make, my level of happiness becomes higher and higher. The amazing news has given me a kind of joy I've never experienced before.

When we started this journey, I asked God to surround me with healing hands and He answered my prayers.

I relive the morning's events over and over with each conversation. I'm like a giddy kid without a care in the world. I feel relief and a sense of accomplishment. Life is perfect and joyful.

Some people cried, and some said, "I knew you could do it."

Dassy told me: "You worked hard to get this result. Not everyone would do what you did. It's much easier to follow the doctor's orders, because then you don't have to think about it."

One friend said: "I am so relieved. I supported you, but all along I was wishing you'd do what the doctors said to do. I'm happy you proved me wrong."

It's overwhelming! I can't find the words to explain the feeling, but everyone is happy and excited.

This is another one of life's defining moments.

Next is a text to Dr. Bartiss: "Holy sh*t bag! Guess who's CANCER FREE? ♥ Paula" It may sound crass, but politically incorrect humor helped me get through this medically trying time. (Those in the medical industry know that sh*t bag is the slang word used as a reference to a colostomy bag.)

Once Jack and I finish our business, we have lunch on the terrace of the Logan Inn. We sit across from each other, with our arms stretched out across the table and holding hands. We probably look like a couple on one of their first dates: totally interested in each other's conversation.

"Is it just me, or is today the absolute most beautiful fall day ever?" I ask as I stare across the table at Jack.

"Everything is picture-perfect. The sky is the bluest blue and just the right amount of clouds." Jack smiles back at me.

Jack orders a salade Niçoise; I have an organic beet salad with fresh raspberry vinaigrette. Our lunch tastes especially good today.

Bartiss calls later that evening, "I cried when I received your text. Tell me everything: How do you feel? How about Jack, Katie and your sisters? How did everyone react when you told them the incredible news?"

He cares; he shares in my amazing joy! Mark's reaction is certainly more normal than that of the conventional doctor who first gave me the fantastic news earlier today.

I recommend Mark James Bartiss, MD, to anyone who appreciates the natural approach to health. Dr. Bartiss is generous with his knowledge and passionate about getting his patients healthy. Patients are treated as individuals, not protocols.

There was never any doubt in my mind that Mark wanted to help cure my cancer. At times, he even had me laughing about my circumstance, which made the situation bearable.

I thank God every day that I had the courage to go against the grain. Seven experts in their fields told me my only option for a cure was a life-changing surgery.

When I felt doubt about my decision, I listened to my inner voice. It always pointed me to people who believed that the body can heal itself.

Meeting Mark was yet another defining moment in my life because it gave me the belief I needed to change my course of action.

I will be forever grateful that God put Mark James Bartiss in my path.

I guess I'll never be sure of what actually took the cancer away. I guess it was everything combined.

Here is a list of all of the different modalities used:
First there was a lot of prayer.
Then came:
Chemotherapy and radiation
Mangosteen juice during chemo
The belief that my body could heal itself
Change of diet
Clean, organic food
Raw milk and yogurt
Creative visualization
Hypnosis
Ozone/ultraviolet infusion
Ozone saunas
Healing massage
Exercise
Crystals
Yoga and meditation
Acupuncture
Compounded hormones
Essential oils
Lots of supplements, such as laetrile(B_{17})
Water from the Lourdes Grotto in France
Life in the Spirit charismatic healing sessions
Pentecostal healing Masses

Self-help courses
Learning to let go
Gratitude
And last but not least, Self-Love.

After a body detoxification, the rest of the healing was spiritual, emotional and psychological.

I give all the glory to God and I thank Him every day that I listened to my intuition.

I'm also thankful to my family and friends who stood by me and supported my decisions during this difficult yet fascinating journey.

Jack and I end the day enjoying the peacefulness of our own backyard. Jack says, "This moment is surreal, and we're living what we dreamed of for the past two years."

"Yeah, the feeling's right up there with falling in love, right up there with giving birth. It's pure joy!"

Now one last follow-up with the oncologist.

Chapter 20   Miracles Happen Every Day

The post cancer visit with Dr. Rivers the oncologist is unremarkable—a term used in the medical industry.

Jack and I are pleasantly surprised that unlike, the other doctors on the cancer team, Dr. Rivers seems very happy for us.

As a member of the cancer team, her job is to talk us into the surgery. From our past meetings, though, the doctor knows that that would be a futile endeavor.

Instead, the conversation is light and jovial.

Dr. Rivers says, "The biopsy report is marked *unremarkable*. All is clear. No malignancies and every biopsy is benign. I recommend a yearly colonoscopy for follow-up to make sure the cancer has not come back."

Dr. Rivers reveals to us: "You have been the talk of the cancer team for the past twenty months. We all thought you were crazy and unreasonable for not following our professional recommendations. This has never happened to me before: you are not normal; you're what we call an anomaly or rarity."

I say, "I'm OK with that—with not being normal."

Even though she's happy with the conclusion, she never inquired about what I did to help myself. Not one of the doctors on the cancer team ever asked what I did to become cancer free. Most, not all, doctor visits are about what meds they can prescribe for a certain condition. The schools are churning out doctors who know more about available pharmaceuticals than they do about true healing practices.

Shortly after getting the great news, I asked myself the same question the Peggy Lee song asks: "Is That All There Is?"

After two years of disappointing PET scans, CAT scans, X-rays and positive biopsy reports, when I received the incredible news that I am now cancer free, something very strong inside me said, *You have to share this.*

I felt I had to *do* something with the information I'd found out. I still have some mental healing to do; once you've had cancer, you always worry about whether it might come back.

Then, at a luncheon with Grace Asagra and Jack, the two of them started talking about how my story would make a good book — especially if Jack contributed a recipe section, because we all feel the healing started in the kitchen. I thought they were joking, but they weren't.

And that's when the seed was planted. Jack thought a book would add to the healing experience by putting in writing what we'd lived through.

Once I realized the endeavor was important to Jack, I was all in.

In my life, I never thought I'd write anything longer than an e-mail! I had never thought of — much less planned on — writing a book; it seemed a crazy idea.

I thought the cancer experience would be one of the chapters in my life I was going to keep to myself. I didn't even want anyone to *know* I had cancer.

I didn't write this book to change people's minds about treatments they're receiving. Certainly, every one of us should make personal decisions when it comes to our healthcare. The goal of the book is to raise awareness about choice and about empowerment through education.

I want people to know it's OK to question their doctors, to think for themselves and to do their own research. No one should allow medical scare tactics to affect their healthcare decision making.

So, listen to your inner voice and heed your intuition.

Be willing to live with the consequences of your choices.
Be patient.
Don't give up – or give in.
It may take time to heal naturally if natural healing is
your choice.

My short-term goal is to connect with a foundation to
help with fundraising. I would like to be associated with
an organization that provides newly diagnosed patients
with funds to pay for initial consultations with alternative-
care or complementary-care physicians.
People need to realize they have choices.

The ultimate goal is that alternative modalities become
eligible for healthcare insurance coverage. One of the
reasons patients don't choose natural alternative healing is
that it's not covered by insurance. And that discussion
could be a book by itself.

In conclusion, when *fear* knocks at the door, let *faith*
answer. You just might find *no one* there.

Miracles happen every day.

All you have to do is BELIEVE!

"I can do all things through Christ, who strengthens
me."
                                    — Philippians 4:13

I cherish that Bible quote. I look at it daily because it's
an affirmation that I've hung next to my bathroom mirror.

It wasn't until I decided to end my book with it that I realized the significance the chapter and verse numbers mean to me. It so happens that on April 13, or 4/13, of 2005, my mother died of cancer.

And my life changed then, also.

I sincerely wish this book gives you hope and strength to change your life for the better.

To My Husband

Everyone's life journey is different.
I'm glad you're with me on this crazy adventure.
Oh, what a ride the past decade has been!
I'm strong because of you; you are my greatest treasure;
and you are a blessing to me.
No words can thank you for all you do for me.
Every day is easier because of you.
You are my everything.
You are my soulmate, playmate, best friend, confidant and
business partner.
My decorator and my handyman, which includes plumber,
electrician,
carpenter, gardener, housekeeper and driver.
My bartender. Ha, my alarm clock! My personal trainer
and yogi master.
My farmer, cook and nurse, or should I say doctor.
You are my support system, my lucky charm, my
sunshine.
You are my very strength.
You're the reason I'm alive today.
I can be myself because you love me as I am.
You lift my spirit; you make me happy, laugh and smile!
You give me courage.
You are always willing to do for others; you are kind,
generous and patient.
You have a heart filled with love.
You are the best thing that has ever happened to me.
I cherish everything about you.
I love you.
Now get some rest, because the next decades are going to
be awesome—just like you!

Resources

Each and every person is unique — and different from each and every other person. Everyone should do individual research. Not every healing method will work the same for everyone, but your personal health is worth the extra time and effort. Following — in no particular order — are some of the Web sites I visited on the Internet, as well as other resources I consulted to do research.

- *The Truth About Cancer: A Global Quest*, a nine-part documentary by Ty Bollinger, who publishes a yearly docuseries. Anyone who receives a cancer diagnosis should check out this series.

- www.chrisbeatcancer.com, a blog about healing cancer by way of nutrition and natural therapies. It's written by chemo-free cancer survivor Chris Wark.

- kriscarr.com: Crazy. Sexy. Cancer. Kris Carr has written great books about juicing.

- Bruce Lipton is in the field of epigenetics, which is fascinating, and he conducts seminars. He wrote the book *The Biology of Belief: Unleashing the Power of Consciousness, Matter & Miracles.*

- I follow Ryan and Teddy, whose Web site is mykidcurescancer.com. You can also follow them on Facebook.

- Cancercrackdown.org is another good source for those who want to heal themselves naturally.

- I researched the Gerson therapy as well as Rene Caisse, who created Essiac tea.

- I read about the Budwig protocol, developed by German biochemist Johanna Budwig in the 1950s, which consists of multiple daily servings of flaxseed oil and cottage cheese, as well as vegetables, fruits, and juices.

- I discovered the Stanislaw Burzynski story. Looking this one up is a must because it's an amazing story. Dr. Burzynski's cancer research and patient care were inspired by the philosophy of Greek physician Hippocrates, part of which was to either help — or not harm — the patient. The modern medical version still implies "First, do no harm." In my opinion, Big pharma renounces Dr. Burzynski because he offers antineoplaston therapy — an alternative cancer treatment — and because he may be cutting in on the pharma industry's profit centers.

- Holistic practitioner Nicholas Gonzalez, MD, of New York is another alternative doctor I like to listen to and watch on YouTube. Dr. Gonzalez was personal physician to Suzanne Somers. Sadly, Dr. Gonzalez passed away unexpectedly in July 2015. He is part of Erin Elizabeth's *Health Nut News Unintended Series*, which covers the 50 or more holistic doctors who have passed away strangely, suddenly and unexpectedly in the past couple of years.

- In *Run from the Cure: The Rick Simpson Story*, a medical marijuana film, Rick shows how he uses hemp plants to make cannabis oil to cure cancer and gives it away free.

Contact Information

Mark James Bartiss, MD
        www.ICAMBartissMD.com
Grace Asagra Stanley, RN-HC, MA
        www.graceasagra.com
Suzette Lucas
        suzettelucas@gmail.com
Charles F. Stueber, DAc, Lac, Dipl. Ac
        www.acupuncturehamilton.com
Paula Plantier
        www.editamerica.com

Please like my Guided Cure page on Facebook for information on juicing, healthy foods and healing naturally.

I can't end this book without thanking two writers' groups: The Hamilton Marketplace Writers Group meets on the first Tuesday of the month at 7 p.m. at Hamilton Marketplace's Barnes & Noble bookstore. The other writers group meets weekly, on Mondays, at 1 p.m. at the Hamilton Free Public Library.

When, at times, I was tempted to toss *Guided Cure's* manuscript into the fireplace, Mark, Dave, and Dennis of the Hamilton group gave me the confidence and courage to continue writing. I thank them for convincing me that *Guided Cure* is a story the world must hear.

The Hamilton library group, led by Rodney, helped me stay on track, with weekly lessons that sharpened my ability to articulate my thoughts into the written word. I am forever grateful to this group for sharing their knowledge and experience with me.

Both writing groups' members will always have special places in my heart. *Guided Cure* wouldn't be the book it is without the support and encouragement I received by attending the groups' meetings.

All of you are blessings to me because I feel God put you in my path.

Made in the USA
San Bernardino, CA
24 January 2018